Beyond Hope

Closing in on the Cure for Cancer

by Diane Karchner

ISBN 978-0-9895633-2-1

Published by Big Hat, LLC
www.dianekarchner.com

Printed by CreateSpace, an amazon.com company.

All Bible verses from New International Version (NIV)

Permission granted to use quotes from the blog wherewegonow.com.

Dedicated to all cancer researchers
who believe there will be
a cure for cancer some day soon.

❀ ❀ ❀ ❀

In Memory of
Dr. Peter J. Corey

1929 - 2013

✽ ✽ ✽ ✽

Introduction

I had cancer in 1973. My cancer was cured.

My sister got cancer in 2007. She was not cured. She died in 2008.

I know both sides of the heartbreak of cancer. I have experienced firsthand the treatment traumas, and I have seen what happens to a family when all hope is lost.

I wrote this book for three reasons…

First, to remember what it was like to have cancer, a memoir of sorts, about a topic I have rarely talked about, even with my family.

Second, I wrote it to bring awareness to where we were and the incredible work of researchers to get where we are now — so much closer to a cure for all cancers.

Most of all, I wrote this to give hope and encouragement to those in the battlefield right now. It was not easy in 1973. It is not easy in 2016.

I surveyed twenty survivors — or those in remission, even some still in treatment. Their quotes and inspiration are peppered throughout the book. Since my experience with cancer is but memories clouded in decades of time, their gracious willingness to provide perspectives helped to ensure I captured the reality of today. Every word they shared is grounded in the experience of a diagnosis that required much to overcome. I am so thankful for their input.

As I am not a medical profession, nor have I ever received any medical training whatsoever (other than a CPR class 15 years ago), nothing in this book should be considered medical advice in any way. I've referenced a few things for those interested in digging into more, but if you are currently on the battlefield, this book is not your medical answer, but will hopefully serve to encourage you in the fight.

Everything in this book is based on what will soon be out-of-date knowledge of cancer, its treatment and its cure rates. Eventually this book will be about the disease that used to be and is no longer.

My prayer is that all its readers will be encouraged, entertained, inspired and filled with hope.

A special shoutout to my always-editor, my husband, who is always my first and last and continuing encourager in all my writing; and to my friend, Jen Thompson, a cancer survival herself who encouraged, edited and connected me with other survivors so I could tell the whole story from 1973 through to today. Thanks to both of you this book was finally birthed!

Welcome to my story!

~~~~~~~~~~~~~~~~~~~~~

Table of Contents

❀ ❀ ❀ ❀

Then and Now

I sat by her bedside holding her hand. She was breathing heavily, air rattling around in her fluid-filled chest. She was bloated and pale, her body puffed and rounded, her skin stretched almost to transparency as the cancer raged through her body. I always imagined near-death being more flat, more concave, sunken. Hers was not.

Her oncologist's words, just a few months before, swirled in my head. *'Since radiation failed, and the last round of chemo failed, we can prolong with a cocktail of several agents. But there is no cure at the end of that round, just a very short remission, possibly, and side effects would be intense.'*

Her words seemed to hang in mid-air as if in a cartoon cloud edged with dark shadows. She left the room while the three of us — my sister, her daughter, myself — processed what she had said. I turned away, leaning my forehead against the cold wall, fighting back the frustration and the utter helplessness. There were no tears. Not yet. On the way home, my sister decided to refuse the chemo. The hospice team came a day later.

This is what cancer almost always looked like in 1973, the year I was diagnosed. Every time a doctor spoke that word to a patient — the "C" word — family life took on a foggy future, suspended in the fear of an early, painful death. Everything became shrouded in that inevitability, foreheads pressed to the wall, trying to find stability from the shifting earth below, trying to get a grip on the new normal. Life was put on hold as death approached.

In 1973, less than 50% of those diagnosed with cancer survived five years. In 2016, there are 14.5 million survivors alive today, with a five-year survival rate of 69% for all cancers combined. Even with those promising statistics, of the 1.6 million new cancer diagnoses that will be delivered this year, over half a million people may still die of it. That is over 1,600 deaths from cancer each day; 1,600 families who will go through the excruciating reality that my family, and many others, did. Every year.[1]

In 1973, I was one of the fortunates, upfront in the line with those who got to bypass this scenario. I was with the many who were given the prognosis beyond remission, to cured. I am so thankful for that and for today's staggering survival rates, appreciation for which is unnoticed until we are touched by the hope of it.

My sister's cancer was called liposarcoma. It has a five-year survival rate of just 16%. Like most cancers in 1973, it carries an almost certain death sentence.[2]

We read so much about leaving a legacy, even writing an idealized eulogy, including   all the seemingly important stuff we think about before we lay bloated and weak on our death bed. It's a good exercise.

[1] http://www.cancer.org/acs/groups/content/@research/documents/document/acspc-047079.pdf

[2] http://www.cancer.org/cancer/sarcoma-adultsofttissuecancer/detailedguide/sarcoma-adult-soft-tissue-cancer-survival-rates

I've done it myself. But sitting by my sister's bed, holding her hand, I realized what a futile waste of time that is. As the end neared, she wasn't thinking about anything that would go into an idealized eulogy of a distant future — stuff that seemed so important before you had only days to live. She thought only about one thing. Her daughter.

She didn't ask me to take care of her daughter, to watch over her, to take her place as the mom. She only said how glad she was that her daughter and I were so close, that she didn't have to worry. It was the only time she saw me cry since her diagnosis, her words cutting through me with blades of sadness.

The truth was that I don't want to be alone with her daughter, or with her granddaughters. I just want to be the crazy aunt who laughs with her, their G-mom. I want my tissue-wrapped presents to be sitting humbly next to her Martha-Stewart-quality wrappings under their Christmas tree. I want to eat her gourmet cooking, not fail miserably at trying to replicate it. I want her to make crafts with her grands like she had done with my daughter. I have been there for her daughter, as much as this crazy aunt can be. But my deepest sorrow remains wrapped in my need to do all of that *with* her.

I was out of town when liposarcoma took her life on April 21st of 2008. Her daughter was there, the hospice nurse close by, taking care, with care, of all the physical-ness of death. I got the call around 9 that night. I phoned who needed to know, then flew home the next morning to the scene of sadness, of finality.

As inevitable as we had feared it would be, in less than a year we had lost the glue that held our extended family lovingly, semi-dysfunctionally, loosely together. In her own obsessive-compulsive way, she was our stability, a label she, and we, would never have used in her life, yet one that became so obvious in her death. An unwelcome, new normal set in all too quickly, too painfully.

Someday, perhaps, this scenario will no longer be. Someday every diagnosis of cancer will end up completely cancer-free, cured. Families will not need to adjust to new normals, with missing faces in the annual family Christmas photos.

But my story did not start with the cure; my story started with a diagnosis that promised nothing.

My story is about the beginning of the end, the hope that there would be a cure for all cancers in the near future.

This book is for all who want to keep that hope alive.

It's nearer than ever before.

~~~~~~~~~~~~~~~~~~~~~

The Isolation of Disease

Fear is one of the main sources of cruelty.

~ Bertrand Russell

As I began to write this, one of the memories that stood out the most was the feeling of isolation. I felt it almost immediately with the diagnosis of cancer and for years after. In today's context, it is hard to believe that those with cancer were treated so much differently in 1973 than the supportive, involved attitudes that prevail today. The best way I could think of to describe the way it used to be is to recall another disease state, easily identified as one of isolation, although for different reasons.

In the 1970s the public began hearing about a new disease, a deadly wasting disease with symptoms as varied as skin rash to sarcomas to immune deficiency which made even a minor cold life threatening. Although cases outside the US were widespread, the first case in the United States wasn't diagnosed until 1981. The following year, the CDC, in collaboration with healthcare organizations around the world, named this disease AIDS: auto-immune deficiency syndrome. In less than a decade this disease had become a pandemic, killing nearly 90% of those afflicted. It was a death sentence.[3]

---

[3] avert.org

Initially, the vast majority of people were so scared of the very thought of the disease that they rejected any interaction at all with those who suffered with it. Could we touch someone with AIDS? Could we be in the same room, use the same bathroom, even breathe the same air? Fear trumped compassion, fueled by the CDC's publication of precautions to prevent "AIDS transmission" and the US government halting immigration of anyone who had it. From 1981 to 1987, of the 50,000 diagnosed with AIDS in the US, 96% died.[4] The gay community, where the disease seemed to be most prevalent, was demonized for their perceived role in causing its spread, adding to the decades of discrimination and prejudice.

The 2013 movie, *Dallas Buyers Club*,[5] was based on the story of Ron Woodruff, who contracted AIDS in 1986, several years before any effective antiviral was on the US market. The story focused on his illegal smuggling of medicines into Texas that helped his 'clients' slow the disease's progress. Using them on himself, he was able to prolong his life for seven years, eventually dying in 1992 of pneumonia, a common complication of the disease. Woodruff's story was a mix of capitalism, compassion, and desperation.[6]

In one of the many heart-wrenching scenes in the movie, Ron walked into his long-time hangout bar where his friends were sitting

---

[4] cdc.gov/mmwr

[5] http://www.imdb.com/title/tt0790636/

[6] biography.com/people/ron-woodruff

around the table with their beers in hand, cowboy boots propped up on nearby chairs. It was the normal place for him to be, Ron greeting everyone as he usually did. But this time his 'friends' did not react in the usual way. They were repulsed at his presence, offended by his nearness, not only because of their prejudiced assumption of his sexuality, but more so of being in proximity to someone with AIDS. They poked fun at him, insulted him, tried their best not to make eye contact let alone touch this infected 'friend'. The scene portrayed a chillingly accurate picture of the effect fear can have on compassion, on friendship. It would be years before this kind of reaction would change.

~~~~~~~~~~~~~~~~~~~

Sickness shows people's true colors.
~Shana, Cancer Survivor

~~~~~~~~~~~~~~~~~~~

At about this same time, cancer was still a deadly diagnosis after decades of taking lives. It carried none of the stigma of questioned sexuality or fears of 'catching it' that AIDS did. It wasn't avoided because it might affect someone's health. But it did repulse, the fear of death lingering heavy in the very air around the word. And because of that, the isolation and loneliness of cancer was just as painful.

I realize in today's world this must be hard to imagine — abandoning a person in the throes of chemotherapy and surgeries and radiation treatments. But that was the way it was in 1973. I know. I was there. I was avoided. Eye contact with passersby was rare. Waitresses didn't look at me when I placed an order. I caught people glancing at me and when I turned to look, they quickly turned away. I was a sideshow, a walking-around sad story to be pitied. Avoidance like that may seem so inconsequential, so minor, yet when your body is destroying itself and your outsides mirror the war zone that is happening inside, being ignored is more than just casual. While I silently screamed for empathy, there was no one tuned into the frequency. No one with ears to hear.

No one wanted to talk about it, to look at my bald head, to ask me questions about the severe nausea. No one wanted to ask me if I was going to live, because in 1973 I probably wasn't going to. I felt alone in the midst of the normal ebb and flow of life. The emotional toll of this kind of isolation is irreversible. It has stayed with me, changed me in ways that are hard to get my head around sometimes.

~~~~~~~~~~~~~~~~~~~~

Let people help you, let them sit with you,
go to your appointments,
and whatever else you need. Ask for help.
You don't need to do it on your own.
~Stacey, Breast Cancer Survivor

~~~~~~~~~~~~~~~~~~~~

The psychological and emotional issues of cancer were not on anyone's radar. No one — the doctors, the caregivers, the nurses — thought about it. In their minds it was doubtful that I would live, so why help with the psychological trauma of isolation or fear of death, or any of it. It just didn't seem to be needed. Not then.

~~~~~~~~~~~~~~~~~~~~~

Don't be afraid to ask people to help you
(meals, childcare, rides, cleaning, etc.).
I found that most friends are very happy to have
a way to help you out.
~Kendra, Cancer Remission

~~~~~~~~~~~~~~~~~~~~~

It was not that others didn't care, that they didn't want to help. I didn't feel unloved by my husband, my family. It's just that people were scared. Unlike the fear of catching the disease as people had with AIDS, they may have been worried about saying the wrong thing, asking the wrong question. They may have been guarding themselves from getting too close emotionally to someone who may be dying. Nearer to the truth would be a recent Harris poll result which found that cancer remains the most feared disease in the US, beating out the disease that actually is the most deadly — heart disease — by more than 30%. It wasn't that they feared catching it from me. They just feared the death sentence attached to it.

Breakthroughs in research and improved clinical outcomes have certainly played a part in altering the perceptions of both AIDS and cancer diagnoses being automatic death sentences.

Avoidance driven by fear is completely understandable in hindsight, but that doesn't make it any easier to accept when you are feeling alone with a disease. Now, fear no longer masks the compassion people have — and show.

There is much understanding, much compassion, and much hope — far-reaching hope — where there used to be none. Beyond remission, straight to cure.

~~~~~~~~~~~~~~~~~~~~

And So It Begins

It was a sunny day in April of 1973. I was twenty years old, married for less than a year. I found a lump in my neck, a little marble under my skin. To me it was more an annoyance than a concern, mostly because it was so visible. It looked kind of like a pimple, so it was vanity that drove me to the doctor thinking he would just get rid of it for me, consumed with the joy of ignorance.

The doctor I saw at the clinic suspected that it was more than a pimple or mole or swollen gland. Hoping it was the not the same thing that he had seen before. His college roommate had the same kind of lump a few years before, with less than a hopeful outcome.

He called the chief of staff at the local hospital, a board member of his clinic, who agreed to see me immediately. So off I went to the hospital to have yet another doctor look at what I still thought was a pimple. He spent less than a minute examining me before he admitted me to the hospital.

I want to believe that fear shook me to the core, that I reacted like any sane person would to being admitted so urgently to a hospital. Maybe I had been, but I don't remember it that way. Instead I remember being highly annoyed by the whole thing. Not because I didn't think it was more than a pimple. I got that. No one gets admitted to the hospital for a pimple. I was annoyed because they didn't tell me what they already knew. When both doctors touched my neck I could tell they knew immediately. I knew that they knew and they wouldn't tell me. And that annoyed me.

In 1973 doctors didn't feel the need to tell their patients much of anything. They had full control of all information channels. They were masters of their universe, holding exclusive rights to any and all medical answers. I was at their mercy and that made me twitchy. Except that when it came to cancer, they were not the infallible lifesavers.

Today an uninformed patient is a rarity. With access to the internet, information — accurate or not — is available to all of us. Medical offices display free brochures for everything from toenail fungus to arthritis exercises. There are ads and pamphlets and websites that can just about put words into your mouth, providing lists of questions to ask a doctor, most of which you would never have thought up on your own. All of this results in an informed patient and a doctor who is forced into a partnership rather than playing all-knowing dictator. It is a win-win.

~~~~~~~~~~~~~~~~~~~~~~

Learn as much as you can about your diagnosis.
Not just from your doctor, but on your own, from reputable sources.
~Kendra, cancer in remission

~~~~~~~~~~~~~~~~~~~~~~

In 1973 the two doctors were my only source of information. They gave me none. If the Internet had existed in 1973, I would have been on it that first day when the doctors told me nothing — what could it be, what was it, what if? After the diagnosis, I would have been all over the staging and the surgeries and the treatment options. But not even the internet would have helped then. There was nothing to report, no information to put on Wikipedia. No nothing — a double negative the best way to describe the vacuum of knowledge at the time. That is except for the dismal survival rates, and who would want to read them?

~~~~~~~~~~~~~~~~~~~~

Ask as many questions as you can.
But be careful not to look too much at
information on the Internet.
Also, everyone's case is different, some
treatments work better for other
people than it would for you. Listen to
your doctors and always try to have a
positive attitude! ~Shelleu, In remission

~~~~~~~~~~~~~~~~~~~~

So, knowing nothing, I went warily into the hospital admissions process and onto my room. Other than being born, this was the first time I had been a patient in a hospital. To me hospitals were a place of birth and death with very little good news in between. That first night no room was available on the surgical floor so I was admitted to the fifth floor, east wing. Every room on the floor was, literally, occupied by someone who was critically ill, who all seemed to have refined the ability to moan at high decibels. And the hacking, mucous-filled coughs! All night. Literally. I dubbed it the Death Wing. It was a Stephen King novel come to life and I was its compassionless, clueless protagonist.

Needless to say, I couldn't sleep with all that clatter so I spent most of that night on the fire escape, in my PJs, wrapped in a blanket, smoking, a full pack done by the time dawn finally burst through. The nurses checked on me from time to time in between addressing the hacking and the bedpans and the plumping of pillows. They came to commiserate and share a smoke or two themselves (it was the 70's!). I am not even sure why I was allowed to sit outside on the fire escape, of all places, but I remember having a great view of the town.

That first night in the hospital, on the Death Wing, I wasn't fearful. I didn't sit on the fire escape because I was scared or nervous. And I didn't sit out there because I was a particularly nicotine-dependent smoker. The pack I inhaled overnight usually lasted me weeks. I was just pissed off. All I was thinking was 'what idiot put me on this floor? If I am going to die, why don't they just tell me? Better yet, kill me now, I can't stand the hacking!' (Oozing with compassion, wasn't I?)

I was moved the next day to the surgical wing, what would soon become my home away from home on and off for the next three months. Even then, I don't remember being all that fearful. Annoyed, yes. Fearful, not so much. Not yet. I was, and still am, an eternal optimist, with little or no filter on what I said and maybe (a big maybe at the time!) a half-smidgen of sensitivity. I was strong-willed and feisty, an iron-fisted, raging feminist of the 70s. And everything was going to be all right. I would beat whatever it was. No worries.

And at that point I still believed that I would live forever. Being twenty had its advantages.

I just wanted to know. Now.

~~~~~~~~~~~~~~~~~~~~

Diane Karchner

❀ ❀ ❀ ❀

The New Field of Oncology

The lump turned out to be a lymph cancer known as Hodgkins Disease then, known today as Hodgkin lymphoma (HL). Make no mistake, whatever its name, it was cancer and in 1973 it was at an all-time 5-year survival rate high of 40%.[7]

At the time of my diagnosis the treatment for cancer, of any kind, fell into the area of hematology. Although approved for inclusion as a sub-speciality in internal medicine in 1972,[8] medical schools had not yet fully developed a specialty track for oncology. There was not yet a board certification available for doctors to specialize in oncology, even if, as my doctor, they were already treating patients with cancer. There were no oncology-specific medical journals to turn to in the library that would have the latest and greatest in cancer research (although Hematology journals did have reports of some of the ongoing cancer research).

Even so, if there was ever a good time to get cancer (and there is never, ever a good time), I was on the cusp of it. Attention to cancer started years before with the passage of the National Cancer Act of 1937 which established the National Cancer Institute (NCI), making it

---

[7] seer.cancer.gov/statfacts

[8] http://jco.ascopubs.org/content/28/22/3653.abstract|

the federal government's principal agency for conducting research and training on the cause, diagnosis, and treatment of cancer.[9]

But it was a woman who really got things going. Her tenacity and dedication, I believe, has led to saving more lives than can ever be counted. The power of a single person, in the right place, with the right heart and conviction, changed the trajectory of even a death sentence like cancer as nothing else could.

Mary Lasker, a New York philanthropist, was one of the country's best known and most effective activists in the cause for increased public funding for medical research. For decades, she tirelessly persuaded the American public that the national investment in medical research would yield invaluable benefits for human health. Her simple warning was, 'If you think research is expensive, try disease!'

"Mrs. Lasker's early efforts focused on developing public support to advance basic research on cancer. She founded the Citizens Committee for the Conquest of Cancer and took her cause to Congress and the American public as a leading proponent of the National Cancer Act, which was signed by President Nixon in 1971."[10] This resulted in a major increase in federal funding ($600M by 1974)[11] specifically targeted to fight cancer. Three comprehensive cancer

---

[9] http://legislative.cancer.gov/history/1937

[10] http://www.laskerfoundation.org/about/legacy.htm

[11] http://cancerprogress.net

centers were immediately designated, charged with translating research results into clinical practice.

Today, the National Cancer Institute (NCI), along with the National Institutes of Health (NIH), fund the work of more than 325,000 researchers at more than 3,000 universities, hospitals, and 66 dedicated cancer centers across the US.[12]

One of those first three cancer centers was the Johns Hopkins Kimmel Cancer Center in Baltimore, a four hour drive from my home. It officially opened its doors with thirteen dedicated faculty members in early 1973, just four months before my diagnosis.[13] For me, my surgeon was the only source for information, for encouragement, for alternative solutions, for anything related to my cancer. If my doctor didn't know, he knew how to make a phone call — to Johns Hopkins — on a landline since there were no cell phones, no Skype, no video chatting.

A doctor. A specialty. A hospital. A landline. If there was ever a good time...

My surgeon became my 'oncologist' in all sense of the word, coached and directed by the researchers and physicians at Johns Hopkins. He removed the lump, did a gaggle of clinical tests, took out my spleen, removed a post-operative cyst, administered two years of

---

[12] http://www.cancer.org/cancer/news/national-cancer-actmarks-milestone

[13] http://www.cancer.gov/research/nci-role/cancer-centers/history

chemo and saw me through ten years of followup exams. The now-mature field of oncology covers all those areas, but in a different way.

Today there are three primary clinical oncology disciplines: medical oncology, surgical oncology, and radiation oncology.[14]

- A medical oncologist specializes in treating cancer with chemotherapy (the use of drugs to kill cancer cells, usually by stopping the cancer cells' ability to grow and divide) or other medications, such as targeted therapy and oral chemotherapy.

- A surgical oncologist specializes in the removal of the tumor and surrounding tissue during an operation. A surgical oncologist also performs biopsies (the removal of a small amount of tissue for examination under a microscope).

- A radiation oncologist specializes in treating cancer with radiation therapy (the use of high-energy X-rays or other particles to kill cancer cells).

Additionally, the general surgery nurse who took such good care of me during all of my stays in the hospital, would today be replaced by an oncology nurse practitioner (NP) who would serve as a patient's case manager. The NP's role can be as varied as the needs of each specific patient: informing a patient of the details about the specific cancer, coordinating care with the oncologists on the team, playing an integral role in care both during and after treatment.[15]

---

[14] Accessed at Cancer.net on 10/22/2015

[15] Galassi A, Wheeler V: Advanced practice nursing: History and future trends. Oncol Nurs 1(5):1-10, 1994.

In a cancer center today, a typical interdisciplinary oncology team might include as many as five oncologists (depending on the type of cancer), a family nurse practitioner, five infusion nurses, two radiation oncologists, a radiation nurse, three radiation technologists, six medical assistants, two adult nurse practitioners focused on clinical trials research, three clinical nurse specialists, two social workers and three scheduling assistants. All on standby to support a patient diagnosed with cancer.[16]

Cancer patients may not actually see all of these team members, but they certainly can be confident that their diagnosis, treatment and followup are backed up by many dedicated oncology-specific healthcare providers.

I had my surgeon.

He had a landline to Baltimore.

~~~~~~~~~~~~~~~~~~~~

---

[16] http://nurse-practitioners-and-physician-assistants.advanceweb.com/continuing-education/cc_articles/nps-in-oncology.aspx

Diane Karchner

❀ ❀ ❀ ❀

Anatomy of a Cancer

A century is only a small segment in the timeline measuring the history of science through the ages. But for cancer research, the last 100 years overshadow all of the years that came before. Physicians have moved from being able to do very little to treat patients to achieving survival and cure rates no one believed possible. Just a few decades ago, young investigators and physicians were often told not to go into oncology because the disease is so complex and the clinical outcomes were so discouraging. Today, oncology is one of the most exciting fields in biomedicine because of the many astonishing advances research continues to yield. [Weinstein IB, Case K. Cancer Res September 1, 2008 68; 6861]

~~~~~~~~~~~~~~~~~~~~

For years I believed cancer was something that had entered my body and just started to grow, and spread. I imagined that an invader had taken residence inside of me and would burst out of me one day, like the little monster that crashed out of the man's stomach in the 1979 movie, *Alien.*[17] Very sci-fi, but in some naive way the sci-fi seemed easier to grasp.

---

[17] http://www.imdb.com/title/tt0078748/

The reality is that cancer is caused by some cells — my own cells — getting screwed up. Within every healthy cell is a process called apoptosis, which is a suicide switch that the cell initiates when it gets old. It dies as another cell is born, and so it goes. No extra cells lurking around. No more. No less. In this way our body stays energized with each cell at peak performance.[18]

Cancer happens when a cell doesn't pull the kill switch. It has a screw - I mean, chromosome — loose and keeps on replicating. On and on, beyond any need for it to do so. A tumor, then, is a mass of my own cells born out of a rogue cell that decided not to follow the rules. This mass then invades the tissue of its birth organ or body location and cancer is born.[19]

A very simplistic view of cancer. Very simplistic.

On a chromosome level, it is a bit more complicated. The American Cancer Society explains it well in this excerpt from their 'History of Cancer.'

Oncogenes: These genes cause cells to grow out of control and become cancer cells. They are formed by changes or mutations of certain normal genes called proto-oncogenes, the genes that normally control how often a cell divides and the degree to which it specializes in a specific function in the body.

---

[18] http://www.ncbi.nlm.nih.gov/pubmed/10688869

[19] http://www.cancer.gov/about-cancer/what-is-cancer#how-cancer-arises

Tumor suppressor genes: These are normal genes that slow down cell division, repair DNA errors, and tell cells when to die. When tumor suppressor genes don't work properly, cells can grow out of control, which can lead to cancer.

It may be helpful to think of a cell as a car. For it to work properly, there need to be ways to control how fast it goes. A proto-oncogene normally functions in a way that is similar to a gas pedal — it helps the cell grow and divide. An oncogene could be compared to a gas pedal that is stuck down, which causes the cell to divide out of control. A tumor suppressor gene is like the brake pedal on a car. It normally keeps the cell from dividing too quickly just as a brake keeps a car from going too fast. When something goes wrong with the gene, for example if a mutation causes it to stop working, cell division can get out of control.[20]

In 1890, Theodor Boveri, a German biologist, made the first link of cancer being caused by genes gone awry. Eighty-five years later, the year I was diagnosed, there were still only minor advances being made towards a cure. Advances were moving at a snail's pace. Today, the time it takes to get from one breakthrough to the next is collapsing. It is collapsing fast. Look at a few — a very few — of the breakthroughs over just the past twenty years.[21]

---

[20] http://www.cancer.org/acs/groups/cid/documents/webcontent/002048-pdf.pdf

[21] http://www.scientificamerican.com/article/mapping-the-cancer-genome/

- In 1993, Gleevec was developed, the first therapy to target a gene-based cause of a rare strain of leukemia.
- In 1995, the BRCA1 gene was identified in women at high risk for an invasive cancer of the breast; a year later, BRCA2 gene was identified. Both have proven essential in the fight against the most aggressive strains of breast cancer.
- In 2002, a mutation of the B-RAF gene was identified that is common to 70% of melanomas.
- In 2006, a vaccine for the prevention of cervical cancer was launched.
- In 2013, editors of Science deemed immunotherapeutic approach, using certain parts of a person's immune system to treat cancer, a "turning point in cancer."
- By 2016, six immunotherapies are on the market for the treatment of various cancers

Nothing helped to accelerate this quickening trend of discovery more than the Human Genome Project. This quickening pace of solutions was inspired by researchers like Renato Dulbecco, a pioneering cancer researcher and Nobel laureate, who reported in the 1986 Science journal:

If we wish to learn more about cancer, we must now concentrate on the cellular genome. We are at a turning point. Discoveries in preceding years had made clear that much of the deranged behavior of cancer cells stemmed from damage to their genes and alterations in their functioning. There are two options.

Either try to discover the genes important in malignancy by a piecemeal approach, or sequence the whole genome.[22]

Nothing helped to accelerate this quickening trend of discovery more than the Human Genome Project, heralded years before its completion as being a crucial component in the war against cancer. Although final results were not published until 2003, its findings started spilling out and getting used at its inception in 1990. In May 2013, Dr. Giulio Draetta, M.D., Ph.D., a professor in the Department of Genomic Medicine and the director of the Institute for Applied Cancer Science at MD Anderson Cancer Center, shared that information obtained from DNA sequencing is affecting cancer research in three main areas.

• *First, mutations that affect cancer cells' sensitivity to treatment have been identified.*

• *Second, genetic information has revealed common themes in cancer cells that explain their resistance to treatment. "Most tumors inactivate certain mechanisms that induce cell death. The tumors tend to survive even if you bang them with radiation therapy or chemotherapy," Dr. Draetta said. "We can develop all sorts of therapies, but there is resistance because tumors don't want to die. Now, at the genome scale, we know that these mechanisms that induce cell death are the predominant mechanisms of resistance that we have to deal with."*

---

[22] http://www.scientificamerican.com/article/mapping-the-cancer-genome/

• *Finally, DNA sequencing has revealed a greater extent of heterogeneity among cancer genomes than was once thought.*[23]

All of that might sound confusing, even mind numbing, but to put it more simply, it means that researchers are getting closer and closer to figuring this out. And no one is giving up.

In early 2016, Vice President Joe Biden, moved by the death of his son from brain cancer in 2015, launched a new initiative bringing attention to the research that will be required to get to the 100% cure. Biden's plan described increased funding, from both the government and the private sector, for combating cancer. He also focused attention on "breaking down silos and bringing all the cancer fighters together—working together, sharing information, and ending cancer as we know it." Calling it his 'moonshot' to the cure, the goal is to double the pace of progress, or as he put it: "to make a decade worth of advances in five years."[24] It really is just a matter of time.

For some, like my sister, like VP Biden's son and like the half million others who are projected to die from cancer in 2016, it's not in time. But it may be in time for the many hanging on in all stages of remission limbo. It may be in time for the millions who will be

---

[23] http://www2.mdanderson.org/depts/oncolog/articles/12/5-may/5-12-1.html

[24] http://www.sciencemag.org/news/2016/01/what-vice-president-biden-s-moonshot-may-mean-cancer-research

diagnosed in the future, who can truly hope of joining the 14.5 million cancer survivors who are living and breathing in the US today.[25]

In 1890 close to zero survived. A hundred and twenty-six years later, 69%[26] survive for more than five years. In 2026, can we dream...?

It's getting close. Really close.

~~~~~~~~~~~~~~~~~~~~

[25] http://www.cancer.org/acs/groups/content/@research/documents/document/acspc-047079.pdf

[26] http://www.cancer.org/acs/groups/content/@research/documents/document/acspc-047079.pdf

Diane Karchner

❀ ❀ ❀ ❀

The Waiters

I always tell the newly diagnosed that it will be harder for their friends and family than it will be for them. As a cancer patient, you know exactly what you need to do to fight it. As a person who loves a cancer patient, you often feel helpless. You want to help the person fight, but the fight is really up to them and their doctor. I tell newly diagnosed people that they may feel as if they have to be the ones to comfort their friends and family.   ~ Kim, Breast Cancer survivor

~~~~~~~~~~~~~~~~~~~~

I never thought much about my family when I was in the throes of surgery and chemotherapy. Maybe it was because I was so young and self-centered, maybe it was because I was just focused on beating it. It was probably a little of both.

My husband used to come to my hospital room every day and sit at the bottom of my bed reading his Wall Street Journal. Sometimes I would be in a mood so foul that I kicked him out, told him to go home. Sometimes I didn't talk at all. But still he came and still he would sit at the end of the bed. Sometimes he brought food to eat, sometimes he picked at what I couldn't eat from the hospital tray.

He always showed up. Always.

I didn't know until years later that after visiting hours were over, he drank a six-pack of beer every night so he could pass out, as sleep was evading him when sober. He often traveled the half hour to his parents' home so he would not have to spend a night alone. He stopped at a local church even though we hadn't attended any church since he was a teenager (other than our wedding day).

He worried non-stop. He is like that. But I didn't see it. He was just himself when he sat at the bottom of the bed. Quiet. Calm. We had only been married a year. I know him now, can sense his moods, his ups and downs. I know now what worry looks like on him. In 1973, all I knew was that he showed up. Every night.

Then at home, for the next two years, when he found me on the bathroom floor after hours of post-chemo retching, he always brought me a blanket. He knew if I hadn't started shivering from cold sweats already, I would shortly.

Showing up.

~~~~~~~~~~~~~~~~~~~~

A cancer diagnosis makes everyone
realize that we are not indestructible.
While I was under treatment, it was wonderful
to see my family and friends
doing what they could do to help.
~Connie, Cancer Survivor

~~~~~~~~~~~~~~~~~~~~

That's what the family does, the ones who wait. In cars, in waiting rooms, in doctor's offices, eating alone, waiting for calls. Silent. Waiting. In 1973, fear was alive and well in the waiters. They had no one to stand by them. There were no cancer support groups, no specialists or nurse practitioners who understood and addressed the needs of the family. No one could tell them how to comfort the sick or the dying. No one could tell them how to cope with a life on hold, how to grieve the possible loss.

~~~~~~~~~~~~~~~~~~~~~~

My husband has been very
supportive but he became
very angry during those years.
We were able to work through it
but it took time. ~Jennifer, Cancer Survivor

~~~~~~~~~~~~~~~~~~~~~~

Today it is different, thanks to organizations like the American Cancer Society. Their Caregivers and Family section on the website begins with: 'A cancer diagnosis affects close friends and family too. Find out what to expect if you become a caregiver for a person with cancer, and get tips for making sure that you take care of yourself as well.' It goes into sections specifically for how to care for someone with cancer, how to take care of yourself as a caregiver, support groups that are available to the family and caregivers, and on and on.[27] This

---

[27] http://www.cancer.org/treatment/caregivers/

upsurge in attention to those who are a part of the life of a person with cancer validates the need for a holistic view of cancer treatment which extends beyond just the patient. It extends to the community in which they live.

Studies indicate that anxiety and depression are prevalent in family members, almost as much as with the patients. A friend of mine, a breast cancer survivor, recently shared with me that her husband suffered a severe anxiety attack while traveling on business after caring for her post-surgery for the previous 10 days. He spent a night in a hospital ER several hours from home, with symptoms so severe that the staff believed he was having a heart attack.

~~~~~~~~~~~~~~~~~~~~~

It was harder on my family and friends.
It has made many relationships
stronger. We found out how blessed
we are with the community of people
that we are surrounded with.
~Stacey, Cancer Survivor

~~~~~~~~~~~~~~~~~~~~~

In a recent study, the National Institute of Health (NIH) reported that 62% of family members experience anxiety about the patient's future; and 48% report deep unhappiness and depression.[28] These findings are certainly not surprising. Yet in 1973 there was no consideration of

---

[28] http://www.ncbi.nlm.nih.gov/pubmed/19187163

any of that for the family members. There was no training for healthcare providers on how to help. It wasn't even an afterthought. Considering that most patients did not make it past five years, hospice care and funeral planning seemed to be the only needs for the family and friends. Harsh sounding, but the cancer world was, and is, a harsh one.

~~~~~~~~~~~~~~~~~~~~~

There is nothing like a cancer diagnosis
to make one feel loved!
However, that all wears off
eventually. ~Stella, Cancer Survivor

~~~~~~~~~~~~~~~~~~~~~

A recent study indicates that families who are able to act openly, express feelings directly, and solve problems effectively have lower levels of depression overall.[29] In 1973 there was no one to be open with, there was no one to express feelings to, and discussing solutions to problems was non-existent. The families just sucked it up and waited.

Worth noting in this change in dynamics between the healthcare providers and the family of a patient, is the role of the nurse practitioner (NP). As mentioned in a previous chapter, the NP takes on the role of case manager for the patient, involving the family as much as it does the patient. One NP described her daily routine as 'support

---

[29] http://onlinelibrary.wiley.com/doi/10.1002/pon.773/abstract]

to patients and their families, advocating for the patient and their families, treating the whole person, not just the cancer.'[30] Cancer treatment is no longer just about diagnosis and research and administering chemotherapy regimens. Now, it includes everyone touched by the disease.

~~~~~~~~~~~~~~~~~~~~~~

Cancer affects more than the patient.
Family and friends rallied.
~Grace, 'currently cancer-free'

~~~~~~~~~~~~~~~~~~~~~~

It is this role that has made the difference in how the waiters wait. Today they still wait. They still show up. But they no longer have to be alone. They have those who will wait with them, who will give them information, who will hold their hand.

The waiters now have others who will show up for them.

~~~~~~~~~~~~~~~~~~~~~

---

[30] http://www.cancer.net/blog/2014-05/spotlight-oncology-nurses

My Doc

It has been four decades since my cancer was cured. As I reflect these many years later, one thing remains. My doctor was the most important partner in my fight. He was not a specialist in oncology, had no published research to brag about, knew little about what to do. Yet he wore his fallibility like a badge of honor. He wasn't sure he could save me, but his actions screamed that he was willing to die trying.

I heard about him before he walked into my room. I was told that the Chief of Surgery had taken my case. I was warned that he was very abrupt, that he didn't do small talk, and he hated 'chatter.' They also told me he was the best.

His name was Dr. Peter J. Corey. On his white surgical coat was embroidered in dark blue script the name "PJ Corey" followed by an alphabet of credentials. At first, I trusted him just because of those letters even though, other than M.D., I had no idea what they meant. I assumed they were attached to some kind of authority, some higher level of education and training and skill. The simplicity of trust based on a mishmash of letters seems absurd, yet it worked for me at the time.

The first time he walked into my room I commented on his embroidery, calling him PJ. The nurse that stood next to him, gasped.

He brusquely corrected me, introducing himself as Dr. Corey, Chief of Surgery. I just grinned at him.

Then he went right to the business at hand, telling me what he was about to do. Cut me open. Take out the lump in my neck. Figure out what it was. Then we will go from there. Without looking at me at all, he jotted something in a big metal chart, slammed it shut, handed it to the nurse, and turned to leave.

I, not so quietly, asked him if I could see the lump after he took it out. (That wanna-be med student in me still lives!) He said no. I said, 'Why not? It's mine.' He had nothing. He just turned and left. I did get to see the lump before it was taken away for study. First battle with PJ, won. I was now the invincible twenty year old. Feisty. No filters. I was prepared for battle, except my foe was so much more ominous than a surgeon named PJ.

~~~~~~~~~~~~~~~~~~~~~~

Take one day at a time, if possible.
Talk to other people, even if every
story is different. Listen to your doctors,
but don't be afraid to ask
questions. ~Kathy, In Treatment

~~~~~~~~~~~~~~~~~~~~~~

For the next five days, I just hung out in a hospital gown and robe, smoking in the lounge, watching daytime TV on one of the only five TV stations in existence at the time. In 1973, my health insurance company had little veto-power over how long I stayed in the hospital, or even how serious my condition had to be to warrant a hospital stay. Decisions were always made by the medical community alone. Health insurance was purchased to cover the expenses that the doctor incurred, and needed little to no justification for payment. It is a far cry from where we are today, with doctors and hospitals under strict scrutiny to adhere to common practices mandated by the insurance companies and the government. For better or for worse, it is different. Today I doubt I would have hung around as a patient in a hospital waiting for a blood test result!

Each morning, PJ, with his bevy of med students marched in and he told me what horror he was going to put me through that day. I always laughed at him, told him he was a masochist, and forced him to tell me what every test was for, in detail. I wanted to know how he thought it would help. I believed in his 'letters', in his credentials, and I put them to the test.

At first, I think I did it to tease, to try to embarrass him in front of his med students. But after a couple days, I bumped up the questions a couple of notches and forced him to give full disclosure of what he thought he would find, what if I didn't have the test, what then? I am certain that most of the questions were much less intelligent than I envision now. But not once did PJ ever act like they were dumb. Not once did he make me feel like a dumb kid who needed to shut up and just follow the rules. I never, ever let him off the hook. Not once. And he never let me down. Not once.

The nurses loved the way PJ and I bantered all the time. It wasn't typical behavior for the big, gruff Chief of Surgery. But after my initial encounter with him, I stopped doing it for that kind of attention. I did it because I wanted him to be real, to not pull a haughty better-than-me bullshit arrogance that would leave me feeling deceived, or angry because I wasn't being told everything.

~~~~~~~~~~~~~~~~~~~~~~

Just wanted to get things moving,
do what I needed to do — surgery, chemo and move on.
~Stacey, Breast Cancer Survivor

~~~~~~~~~~~~~~~~~~~~~~

After a painful bone marrow extraction, a weird lymphangiogram that turned my feet blue, X-rays of every part of my body, and gallons of blood sucked out of me, PJ delivered the verdict. Hodgkin lymphoma. Cancer. It was serious yet it was a relief. At least we could do something other than stick me with needles. We could make decisions. We could get me out of the hospital. But it wasn't going to be so easy. And it was far from the last time I would see the inside of a hospital.

Five years later, when chemo was done and remission tentatively confirmed, he released me from his care. I remember that day, and our conversation, on what we called my graduation. We both had tears in our eyes. My hair had grown back. I was back to a healthy fighting weight. I no longer looked like a cancer patient.

~~~~~~~~~~~~~~~~~~~~~

I got to business to try and find out the
extent of it and what my treatment plan could be.
I treated it as I would a cold, it was a
nuisance, a "breast thingy", not cancer.
~Nancy, Breast Cancer Survivor

~~~~~~~~~~~~~~~~~~~~~

He told me that five years before he thought he would be attending my funeral, not my graduation. We still didn't know if I could have kids. No one thought I could. But then they also thought I would lose all my teeth by the time I was thirty.

I still have all my teeth (except one). And two years after that graduation, I brought our first child to meet him. I pretended that I named him PJ just to see him squirm with emotion. It worked. He did, that big ole wuss of Surgery!

I believe he was the first live teddy bear I had ever met.

I will never forget him.

~~~~~~~~~~~~~~~~~~~~~

Diane Karchner

❀ ❀ ❀ ❀

Blood Tests and X-rays

Biopsy the lump. Done.

Diagnosis: Hodgkin lymphoma (HL)

Next step: Determine what stage the cancer was in; that is, how far had the cancer progressed. Treatment could not start until the cancer was staged.

Knowing how far the cancer had spread was crucial in choosing the right treatment regimen. In 1973, there were four diagnostic tools at our disposal: X-ray, blood tests, bone marrow extraction and lymphangiogram. All helped determine how far the cancer had spread. Each test added a piece toward solving the puzzle.

The X-rays showed the solid tumors. Three that they could see in my chest, a couple more around my neck. The one that bothered the doctors the most was the larger one in my chest, dangerously close to my right lung and heart. Growth in that one could put pressure on vital organs that could slow treatment, increase the likelihood for complications, and more, although they could not predict anything for sure.

The blood test would indicate two things. In 1973 the doctors knew that a low white blood cell count would indicate a problem and the possibility of higher than usual susceptibility to infection. The doctors also knew to look for an antigen in the blood that had been identified in research as a 'marker' for cancer, especially for leukemia, lymphoma and myeloma.[31] Beyond that, there was little else that would help with staging. Eventually the simple blood test would become a powerful tool in the oncology field, but in 1973 there was still so much to learn.

I then had a bone marrow extract. The most painful of the four, it was also the most vital. One of the criteria for staging a lymphoma was to determine if it was solid tumors or blood-based. Abnormalities in the bone marrow would have caused concern about the extent of the cancer spread. Fortunately, my bone marrow was clear, there were no cancer markers in my blood, my white blood cell count was not too abnormal and the X-rays confirmed some solid tumors.[32] All pointed to an early stage.

Rarely used today, the doctor did try one test called a lymphangiogram[33]. The test was to assess any blockage in the lymph system which runs all over the body to remove waste, deliver oxygen, cool the body. The technician stuck tiny needles between my toes which were hooked up to long tubes that were attached to a crazy looking machine. The objective was to pump some blue dye all through my body that would light up and show them the way to any cancer. Simplistic explanation, but you get the idea. The problem was that the

---

[31] http://www.annclinlabsci.org/content/4/5/323.full.pdf

[32] AJCC 1stEd Cancer Staging Manual, 1977

[33] https://www.nlm.nih.gov/medlineplus/ency/article/003798.htm

tiny lymph capillaries in my feet kept collapsing, backing up the tubes, and pumping the blue dye all over my feet rather than into my body.

Instead of seeing cancer, I ended up with Smurf-blue feet and nothing lit up inside my body except my big toes. Lymphangiogram is rarely used today,[34] replaced by the more advanced radiologic tools available now. So there will be very few patients walking around with blue feet which, by the way, stayed that color for months!

Today cancer patients are put through much more rigorous testing with much more accurate diagnostic tools available to the doctors: CBC blood test, blood protein testing, tumor marking test, and radiologic screenings.[35]

I went home after all the tests, waiting to hear what the next steps would be. The tests had been inconclusive, so we still did not know the extent of the cancer in order to stage it appropriately. Today an MRI, perhaps a CT-PET scan, a couple of tiny incisions to biopsy a tumor or two would be the next steps. In 1973 nothing existed that would come close to the near-conclusive results all of those can provide.

In 1973 there was an X-ray machine, a blood marker, and bone marrow extraction (and blue feet).

The first scan of a human by an MRI machine wasn't done until 1977 and widespread use as a diagnostic tool didn't happen until the late 80's. MRI is not a photograph, but rather a computerized image of

---

[34] http://theoncologist.alphamedpress.org/content/1/1/41.full

[35] http://www.mayoclinic.org/diseases-conditions/cancer/in-depth/cancer-diagnosis/art-20046459?pg=1

the radio signals that are given off by the human body. Today, it is the procedure of choice for healthcare practitioners seeking to see soft tissue images. Since it uses no radiation, just radio waves, the potential for harm is low.[36]

Today, for cancer, the MRI can be used to[37]:

•Find a tumor

•Determine, in some situations, if a tumor is cancerous

•Learn more about the stage of cancer (the size and location of the tumor)

•Help doctors plan cancer treatments, such as surgery or radiation therapy

•Monitor a tumor's response to treatment

A CT, computed tomography, is a "computerized X-ray imaging procedure in which a narrow beam of X-rays is aimed at a patient and quickly rotated around the body, producing signals that are processed by the machine's computer to generate cross-sectional images—or 'slices'—of the body. These slices are called tomographic images and contain more detailed information than conventional X-rays. Once a number of successive slices are collected by the machine's computer, they can be digitally 'stacked' together to form a three-dimensional image of the patient that allows for easier identification and location of

---

[36] http://www.teslasociety.com/mri.htm

[37] http://www.cancer.net/navigating-cancer-care/diagnosing-cancer/tests-and-procedures/magnetic-resonance-imaging-mri

basic structures, as well as possible tumors or abnormalities."[38] Wow, right?

Invented in 1972 by Godfrey Hounsfield of EMI Laboratories, England and Allan Cormack of Tufts University, Massachusetts, the first CT scanners were not installed until 1974. The original systems were dedicated to head imaging only, but "whole body" systems with larger patient openings became available in 1976, with wide distribution by 1980.[39]

A positron emission tomography (PET) scan is a type of imaging test which uses a radioactive substance called a tracer to look for disease in the body. A PET scan shows how organs and tissues are working.[40] One of PET's most significant contributions to health care is in the area of reducing the costs associated with treating cancer by eliminating the need for unnecessary surgeries. Additionally, PET can provide a method of monitoring metabolic response to treatments such as chemotherapy and radiation therapy.[41]

The two scans together — CT and PET — help to stage the cancer, but also can find the exact place to biopsy, assess how the cancer is reacting to treatment, and to pinpoint the most appropriate target for

---

[38] http://www.nibib.nih.gov/science-education/science-topics/computed-tomography-ct

[39] http://www.imaginis.com/ct-scan/brief-history-of-ct

[40] https://cancerstaging.org/references-tools/Pages/What-is-Cancer-Staging.aspx

[41] Maisey NR, Hill ME, Wcbb A et al. *Eur J Cancer* 2000;36:200–206

radiation therapy. The two together have proven to be a combination diagnostic and treatment tool.[42]

Today all of these tools help to determine where the cancer is, where it is not, and give accurate direction to treatment strategies, all available to the entire medical team with a click of a mouse or a touch on a computer screen.

In 1973 there was no touch on a screen or click of a mouse (which was only a furry rodent at the time). Heck, the fax machine was barely in widespread use in 1973.[43] Instead, the records were photocopied and delivered to Johns Hopkins: that is, someone got in a car, paper-based physician notes in hand, blood and tissue samples in an ice chest on the front seat, X-ray films in large brown envelopes, and drove the four hours to the research hospital in Maryland. Then everyone got on the phone — on the landline — to talk about what they could see in my body.

The tests were still inconclusive. The cancer could not be staged with all the data, limited as it was, that made the car ride to Baltimore.

Turned out that for me, in 1973, the only solution the doctor had left was with a scalpel.

~~~~~~~~~~~~~~~~~~~~

---

[42] http://www.cancer.net/navigating-cancer-care/diagnosing-cancer/tests-and-procedures/positron-emission-tomography-and-computed-tomography-pet-ct-scans

[43] http://www.faxswitch.com/fax_machine_history.html

Setting the Stage

Hodgkin lymphoma, as with every cancer, has to be staged. That is, there needs to be a determination about how far the cancer has spread. Whether it is 1973 or 2016, the oncology team needs to know what they are dealing with before hitting a patient with treatments that could do more harm than good if administered needlessly.

First developed in the 1940s, a staging system now known as TNM was developed. It was accepted and refined in 1982, incorporating other staging systems that had been used in different parts of the world. This consistency in language and staging criteria made it easier for clinical and treatment strategies to be identified, shared, and studied. The TNM Staging System became a kind of shorthand way to describe **T**umor growth, the extent of **N**odes involved, and the **M**etastasis (spread) of the cancer.[44]

In 1977 the American Joint Committee for Cancer Staging (AJCC), sponsored by the American Cancer Society (ACS) and National Cancer Institute (NCI), published a comprehensive report based on the TNM Staging System, adding extensive patient intake criteria and diagnostic markers for dozens of different cancers.

---

[44] https://www.google.com/search?client=safari&rls=en&q=history+of+TNM+staging
ı system+for+canccr&ic−UTF 8&oe-UTF-8

Updated regularly (last edition was in 2009; next one expected in 2016), the AJCC report has become the gold standard for cancer patient management. It has enabled all cancer types to be discussed in the same way, while still differentiating the treatment strategies for each stage within each cancer type.[45]

Research in 2000 confirmed that the "proper classification and staging of cancer will allow the physician to determine treatment for the patient more appropriately, to evaluate results of management more reliably, and to compare statistics reported from various institutions more confidently."[46]

From all diagnostics available to the doctors in 1973, it appeared that my cancer was in Stage 2. There was no way to be sure without looking at my spleen, a big lymphatic organ located in the upper left abdominal cavity of my body. The spleen filters the blood, recycling old red blood cells, storing platelets and white blood cells for future fights against infection, like pneumonia and meningitis. It's an organ we can live without (I have for forty years), but since the all-important liver picks up the slack when the spleen is removed, its absence becomes a necessary point of concern when illness comes.

Since there is spleen involvement in up to 40% of lymphomas, confirming the presence of cancer becomes crucial to determining next

---

[45] https://cancerstaging.org/references-tools/deskreferences/Documents/AJCC6thEdCancerStagingManualPart1.pdf

[46] https://cancerstaging.org/references-tools/deskreferences/Documents/AJCC1stEdCancerStagingManual.pdf

steps.[47] Presence of cancer in the spleen would indicate that the cancer would be in either Stage 3 or 4. This was not just an exercise in mapping out the cancer in my body. Stage 2 treatment — chemo only — differed greatly from Stage 3 or 4 treatment — chemo plus radiation. The stronger the treatment protocol, the more damage there could be to the healthy organs in my body, and the longer it would take for the body to bounce back from. In 1973, there were no add-on medicines to help my body's immune system bounce back quickly from the onslaught of poisons being introduced into my body to kill the cancer.[48]

Today, the medical team would have done one of two things to assess the spleen involvement. A tumor might show up on a PET or CT scan, which would be conclusive that there was cancer present in the organ. Not seeing a tumor in the spleen, they would then do a needle biopsy of the spleen, shaving off a sliver of cells or tissue and taking a look, just to make sure.

Early biopsies of the spleen used to hold high risk of bleeding, causing the medical team to often opt for splenectomy — that is, surgical staging — to determine the presence of cancer. Even that risk has been reduced with the advent of fine gauge needles in biopsy

---

[47] Tam A, Krishnamurthy S, Pillsbury E P. et al. Percutaneous image-guided splenic biopsy in the oncology patient: an audit of 156 consecutive cases. J Vasc Interv Radiol. 2008;19(1):80–87

[48] https://cancerstaging.org/references-tools/deskreferences/Documents/AJCC1stEdCancerStagingManual.pdf

procedures. It is rare today to hear of splenectomy being used to stage cancer.[49]

It wasn't rare in 1973 when X-rays were the only radiology tool available, and the amazing translucency of ultrasound and PET scans were years away.

There was only the scalpel.

~~~~~~~~~~~~~~~~~~~~~

---

[49] J Sammon, et al. Image-Guided Percutaneous Splenic Biopsy and Drainage. Semin Intervent Radiol. 2012 Dec; 29(4): 301–310

The Scars and the Detours

Today, with the radiologic tools available, surgery has become, for many cancers, a part of the treatment, part of what goes into beating the cancer. In 1973, for lymphomas in particular, surgery wasn't just a part of treatment. It was also part of the diagnosis, the path that would eventually, hopefully, lead to the treatment decisions.

In 1973, my cancer was confirmed by a lumpectomy of the lymph node in my neck. To determine the stage, they also had to take a look at my spleen. The only way to do that was to do a laparotomy — a surgical staging — of my spleen. Not to be confused with today's bikini-line laparoscopic surgery, this was major surgery with an incision from breastbone to navel, with added holes around the incision for 'drainage'.

The idea of staging Hodgkins lymphoma by laparotomy was only demonstrated as successful in early 1973 — just months before my diagnosis — by John Ultmann and Donald Ferguson of University of Chicago Cancer Research Center. [50] Today this surgery would not be needed, as needle biopsy would have done the trick. Easy peezy.

But nothing was easy in 1973. Instead of an itty bitty needle taking a few cells, the whole spleen needed to come out. They took it out. Finding it free of cancer — meaning Stage 2 — the path forward

---

[50] http://cancer.uchicago.edu/docs/TimelineUCC_17x22Rev913%20FINAL.pdf

became a little clearer. Stage 2 treatment protocol, at the time, was chemo only. This was a good thing. They were as confident of positive results as you could be in 1973. Ten days after surgery, I went home to heal so chemo could begin.

My surgeon did not share anything about his expectations, my chances at survival. He shared the next step forward. He was holding things close to the vest because he knew, for me, that I had hope beyond his words, beyond his incision. He knew giving me information that might prove to be untrue — that might end up as a part of the data of the uncured — would mean I would lose hope. And he knew that hope might be the key to keeping me alive, to keep me fighting.

Three weeks later I was back in the hospital again. Before I could fully recover from the splenectomy, I developed a post-surgical cyst that completely blocked my large intestine. I was full of crap, literally. By the time I checked into the hospital, the intestine had burst and my body, already compromised from the first surgery, was now inundated with the cesspool backup. Back to surgery I went. This time, it wasn't so easy. My body was broken. I was in big trouble. And the doctors didn't have to tell me that. I knew.

I was rushed into surgery on July 4th of 1973 to remove a part of my bowel that had ruptured. That was the easy part. Now I had a shorter intestine, no spleen, and the tumors were still growing in my chest.

The doctors had no idea if the ruptured bowel would affect the cancer growth in a negative way. They had no idea if just opening up my body would cause the cancer to spread or slow down. They had no idea if this infectious onslaught would negate the effects of chemotherapy or even result in unexpected, unknown complications. They just had so little knowledge to go on.

I was in the hospital for the next three weeks recovering. It took them four days to get my fever down and seven more for me to recover enough strength to start harassing the doctor again. My scars were now beyond bikini-banning. They were wider and deeper and darker. They hurt then and still ache from time to time some forty years later. When your body is battered, when it is cut open and the inside places are touched or jabbed or poked or sliced in ways and places they should not be, it is a remembered trauma.

And treatment had not even begun.

~~~~~~~~~~~~~~~~~~~~

Diane Karchner

❀ ❀ ❀ ❀

Mourning the Loss

Cancer always carries scars. For me, as for most, there are visible scars on my body, tracks of things taken, shadows of things that used to be. The memory of the taking eventually dissipates. But as with every loss, no matter what level or depth or traumatic impact, it must be grieved, faced head on at some point and accepted for its absence.

What they took from me I would never get back. It sounds so melodramatic — mourning a spleen, an organ that no one saw anyway. It seems more fitting to be mourning the loss of breasts, of fingers and toes, of a lung or a kidney. Vital, all of them, for self-image and breathing and overall health and wellness. But a spleen?

While researching this book, I tripped upon a heartfelt blog, written by a cancer survivor. I was initially taken back by what she called 'cancer one-upmanship,' but as I thought more about it, I realized that I have often felt that same feeling over the years. There were moments when I thought, 'hey, I've been through so little compared to others.' I had bouts of guilt, triggered by my distaste for talking at all about my cure.

The question of why I am here and healthy, when others are not so fortunate, is painful to ponder. I know that by feeling bad about not suffering enough, I am experiencing "survivor's guilt." But this wise cancer-surviving blogger cleared this up for me. I identified with how she talked about the guilt of the cancer not being worse than it was. This blogger put my feelings into words much better than I have ever been able to.

Survivor's guilt has an ugly cousin. When I experience survivor's guilt I am doing it to myself. When others inflict their judgment upon me that I have not suffered enough, that's survivor's one-upmanship. The truth is that cancer is not a competition and, just as I am enough, so is my cancer. I certainly did go through less than someone else might have gone through. Thank God for that. For that I should be grateful, not made to feel, by myself or anyone else, that I am guilty of not suffering enough to qualify in the cancer games.[51]

The "cancer games." As if we enter voluntarily and choose to play.

"Cancer one-upmanship." As if we would want to 'win' by having gone through a more hellish nightmare than the next person.

Loss is loss and no one can, nor should, judge the level or degree of loss a person feels when something is gone, never to return.

Elisabeth Kübler-Ross, grief researcher and author of the 1969 book *On Death and Dying*,[52] found the process of grief applies to more than just the loss of a loved one, that we indeed grieve the loss of many things from a bad haircut to a wrecked car to a job change.

---

[51] http://www.wherewegonow.com/debbies-blog/cancer-survivors-guilt-its-ugly-cousin

[52] http://www.amazon.com/On-Death-Dying-Doctors-Families/dp/1476775540?ie=UTF8&keywords=on%20death%20and%20dying&qid=1460556060&ref_=sr_1_1&sr=8-1

Kübler-Ross confirmed each of us grieves in our own way: not necessarily for the same kinds of things, not necessarily like anyone else, not even necessarily following along the usual progression of grief.[53]

~~~~~~~~~~~~~~~~~~~~

Since my perspective on life changed
my relationships became more
meaningful and genuine with my family
and friends. I did experience some
painful letting go of friends and a few
distant family members who were
not healthy for me to be around.
~Cathy, Cancer Survivor

~~~~~~~~~~~~~~~~~~~~

Ten years after this spleen surgery I had to have a tooth removed. It was a simple extraction. No big deal. Yet I had the very same sensation of loss as I had after my spleen was removed. I had lost something that I would never get back. It was mine, dang it, and I wanted it back. It was such a strange reaction to something so simple. Who knows if I would have grieved the loss of a tooth at all if I hadn't had cancer, if I hadn't lost so much under the surgery scalpel. But I did, and I do.

---

[53] https://www.psychologytoday.com/blog/thriving-in-the-face-trauma/200910/grief-doesnt-come-in-stages-and-its-not-the-same-every

God created this miracle of a human body and put stuff inside it that should stay in there. I want my spleen back. I don't like having dirty blood or a lymph system that goes awry when it's supposed to be cooling off and cleansing the toxins from my body. I don't want deep, ugly scars all over my stomach. I don't want them to ache when the weather changes.

~~~~~~~~~~~~~~~~~~~~~

In some cases it strengthened my relationships
but with some I feel it changed it, some people treat me different.
~Shelleu, In Remission

~~~~~~~~~~~~~~~~~~~~~

For many cancer survivors loss is what hangs on the longest. Even as we heal, even as we are thankful for being alive, there is a grief. We have lost hair or spleens or breasts or kidneys. Of course, we may have lost the cancer, but that is not a loss. That's a victory. We grieve what we gave up in the process of its destruction.

Thankfulness eases the grief, but it doesn't negate it. And it shouldn't. Loss must be dealt with, otherwise it becomes an unhappy presence, a shadow in your life that seems to haunt more than heal.

Grief is so very personal, not only in what we grieve but in how we do it. Even how long it lasts and if it returns. Just as cancer has its own way of personally impacting our life in different ways. All the loss that goes with its cure is grieved in personal, highly individualistic ways as well.

And grieve, we must.

I know my loss is also my gain, the price my body paid for healing. The scars which scream of my loss are also the proof that I survived, that I beat what most thought couldn't be beaten, what many don't survive even today. My scars tell me, every time I see them in the mirror, that I am a survivor, a fighter, and that my loss was worth it.

But I still miss my spleen. I do.

~~~~~~~~~~~~~~~~~~~~

Diane Karchner

❀ ❀ ❀ ❀

The Birth of Drugs

I have not failed. I've just found 10,000 ways that won't work.
~Thomas Edison

Drugs are discovered in many ways. Many times they come out of the imagination of gifted scientists and researchers, often after years of failure and experimenting, and beginning over and over — *finding 10,000 compounds that won't work*. The development of a drug is not a short one. The time to development is reflected in the costs; but for cancer, it is also reflected most painfully in the number of lives lost as the science progresses and overtakes the death toll.

Prior to 1962, it took a manufacturer about two years to develop a new drug after the molecule was identified.[54] Today, it may take as long as ten years for it to be available to patients, added onto the years of discovering the right molecule, with costs upwards of $500M.[55]

Before the early 1960s, drug manufacturers were under very loose administration and oversight. It wasn't until the thalidomide tragedy of 1961 that the FDA become more involved in the requirements and approval process for drug approval. Thalidomide, a non-barbiturate sedative, was never approved in the US; however, it was available in

[54] http://www.fdareview.org/05_harm.php

[55] Pharmaceutical Research and Manufacturers of America Publication. 21 December 2000. Available at http://www.phrma.org.]

forty-six countries until March of 1962 when it was banned across the world due to its harmful effect on unborn babies.[56]

It was this tragedy that gave the FDA more powerful regulatory authority with the passage of the Kefauver-Harris Drug Amendments Act in 1962, which requires a manufacturer to demonstrate greater safety of the drug before it can be marketed. We take this for granted today, but it was seen as revolutionary in 1962.[57]

But with less risk of harm came more time to get a drug developed and approved, requiring three phases, and much more time, to get approval. Each phase requires years of research and testing before the drug is even presented for FDA approval.

Once a compound has shown some promise of effectiveness, Phase 1 begins.[58] Phase 1 is all about safety with only 10-20 patients being included in the study. On average, only 2/3 of all compounds make it past this phase. Phase 2 increases the number of patients to several hundred. This phase determines the proper dosing (seeking the smallest dose to achieve maximum effectiveness), confirms the most effective method of drug delivery into the patient (IV, oral, etc), and reconfirms the safety established in Phase 1.[59]

---

[56] https://helix.northwestern.edu/article/thalidomide-tragedy-lessons-drug-safety-and-regulation

[57] Hilts PJ. Protecting America's Health: the FDA, Business, and One Hundred Years of Regulation. New York, NY: Alfred A Knopf; 2003

[58] http://www.fda.gov/drugs/resourcesforyou/consumers/ucm143534.htm

[59] http://www.fda.gov/ForPatients/Approvals/Drugs/ucm405622.htm

Up to two years later, depending on length of time for each of the previous phases, Phase 3 begins. Best known as 'clinical trials,' this phase involves the largest number of patients, across multiple clinical sites, with the exact same protocols. This phase takes anywhere from two to ten years depending on the systemic effect of the drug (i.e., how does it affect the heart, lung and liver). Any one clinical trial has multiple sites, but the exact same FDA-approved protocols and criteria for execution. A patient involved in a clinical study is closely monitored per the guidelines of the trial. A patient can't miss a dose, an appointment, a scan. Nothing. All are done according to the criteria laid out in the trial documents.

All clinical trials are maintained in an FDA database of ongoing, planned and completed trials.[60]

The ClinicalTrials.gov website provides current information about clinical research studies to patients, their families and caregivers, health care professionals, and the public. Each study record includes a summary of the study protocol, including the purpose, recruitment status, and eligibility criteria. Study locations and specific contact information are listed to assist with enrollment.

For my sister, after failure on radiation and two rounds of various chemotherapies, our family was introduced to the hope of a clinical trial for a new agent for liposarcoma that was showing some promise. Our family had a hard time grasping the concept of the stringent

---

[60] clinicaltrials.gov

consistency in clinical studies across sites, thinking that moving my sister to a more famous, a bigger, hospital would improve her chances. In reality, it didn't matter if she was enrolled in Philadelphia, Baltimore, New York City or Cleveland. The study was the same. The treatment was the same. The drug was the same.

My sister's hospital was one of the study sites for the clinical trial. She could go through the regimen in the same place where she had been through her whole battle, under treatment by the same oncology team. Not only did it work logistically, but we found out in the process that her oncologist was an international leader in research for my sister's type of cancer. So we had been in the right hands all along. If this cancer could have been stopped, this was the oncologist who would have done it.

Sadly, as we experienced, clinical trials do not always lead to a cure for those enrolled in them. Sometimes, particularly in hard-to-treat diseases, a clinical study becomes a last resort, as it was for my sister. But the cost to do them — in both lives and money — will eventually pay off and lead to a drug, a dose, an idea that will lead to success.

The data from my sister's experience with that drug will, hopefully, be part of the eventual cure. It wasn't in time for her, but it could be in time for others.

Clinical studies are the pathways to the cures.

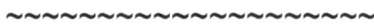

~~~~~~~~~~~~~~~~~~~~

Just a Little More Chemo

It is October 1974. It is the fourth Wednesday of the month. I have been here, in this waiting room twenty-three times before, twice a month, two Wednesdays a month, waiting for an injection of poison.

It is my last dose of chemotherapy for treatment of my cancer, and I am beyond myself with excitement. My last injection. No more hours of nausea, shivering on the bathroom floor. No more weakened immune system which brought every cold and virus that circulated in the air. No more weekly blood tests from scarred veins to make sure my white blood cells weren't attacking any more than usual. My husband and I had planned a celebration for that weekend, a few days after treatment so my stomach could reach a food-welcoming normal, the dull headache gone.

The nurse ushered me into the doctor's office, the doctor who had been through all of this with me from day one. He had operated on me several times, held my hand countless times when pain meds didn't work fast enough, when bandage removals ripped my bruised, thinned skin apart. He was my partner, and my advocate, and my doctor.

When he walked in, he didn't hold the usual little bottle of tablets of the killing compound, or the vial of saline to dissolve the tablets into. He didn't have the syringe in his hand. I thought for an instant that he decided I didn't need this last dose. I was jumping inside my skin with excitement. Until I looked at his face. It was sad, no smiling eyes, no celebration pending. I felt it in my bones this was not going to be a good time. He wasn't joking.

He had just been on the phone with the researchers at Johns Hopkins, reporting my progress, reviewing the latest test results. The same call he had made every month for the past year and a half. They advised that, based on their research and clinical experience with other patients that I should continue the chemotherapy for another year. Another 24 doses. Another year of weekly blood tests on collapsed vessels that bruised with just a touch. Another year.

'Just a little more, Diane. Just a little more.'

His kind words helped me to start breathing again. It was the first time I cried in front of him. In eighteen months I had kept it together, I had been the brave young woman who was going to beat this. I was going to win. Until it felt, just for that moment of breathlessness, I wasn't.

Everyone who has experienced cancer has had a day — or maybe many — like that. Maybe it's a recurrence of the cancer after a year of 'no evidence of disease.' Maybe it's like my sister who needed more than anyone could give. Maybe it's like me, expectations dashed, still more to fight.

In 1973, there was little known about the most effective length of treatment. Researchers were still trying to put some protocols together they could trust. My data would be added in with all the others who sat in their doctor's offices, hoping for good news, but instead receiving the 'just a little more' news.

Chemo for the treatment of Hodgkin lymphoma was based on a drug called mustargen, known in World War 1 as liquid mustard gas. Its chemical name is mechlorethamine hydrochloride, or nitrogen mustard. Used as early as 1915 as a chemical weapon, mustard gas was sprayed into the air, its purpose to slow the enemy down or kill it altogether. Gas masks were completely protective as the affected site could be anywhere on the body. Wherever the gas — actually large crystals — touched the skin it would burn and blister severely. If inhaled, it would burn out the mucous membranes in the bronchial tubes causing respiratory issues that could last a lifetime.

Its effect is best described in this excerpt from a 1918 poem by Wilfred Owen:

> *Gas! GAS! Quick, boys!—An ecstasy of fumbling*
> *Fitting the clumsy helmets just in time,*
> *But someone still was yelling out and stumbling*
> *And flound'ring like a man in fire or lime.*[61]

It was noted by doctors during the treatment of soldiers who had been exposed to mustard gas that their white cell counts were at dangerously low levels. Additionally, those exposed to it showed a suppression of the lymphatic system and an unusual bone marrow effect. At about the same time, a group of civilians in Spain who were

---

[61] http://www.poetryfoundation.org/poem/175898

inadvertently exposed to the gas confirmed all of those same symptoms. With these two diverse populations — soldiers and civilians — the medical community made the connection and theorized that an intravenous application of mustard gas just might kill cancer cells. In a comprehensive overview of the history of chemotherapy, Naomi Elster wrote:

> *And so chemotherapy was born. Like war, it was dangerous and unpredictable, sometimes advancing, often forced to retreat. The first time a patient was treated with cyclophosphamide, the active part of nitrogen mustard, the tumor shrank — something not even thought possible at the time. But it was a temporary miracle. Treatment had to be stopped when the patient's side effects became life-threatening in themselves.* [62]

Eventually they figured out how to dose it appropriately. As the words of Kelly Clarkson's song[63] had it right: 'what doesn't kill you makes you stronger.' By 1949, they had solved the dosing problem and mustargen (mechlorethamine) became the first compound approved for the treatment of cancer — specifically, Hodgkin lymphoma.

By 1965, it made its way into a combination of chemicals — called MOPP (mechlorethamine, vincristine, procarbazine and prednisone) — which became the standard treatment for Hodgkin lymphoma, making it one of the first cancers with improving survival rates.

---

[62] https://www.theguardian.com/science/blog/2014/oct/08/chemotherapy-world-war-cancer-mustard-gas

[63] https://youtu.be/Xn676-fLq7l

Enter me, 1973. I was started on the MOPP regimen as soon as I recovered from the surgeries. That day in my doctor's office seems like just another day in my story, yet when I wrote it the first time, I cried. I cried because I felt, just for a moment, the loss of hope. That it would never end. Or at least not end well. I cried because my sister hoped until the last few days when the morphine wiped hope away. I cried because there are still others going through this, in a bigger more profound way.

For me, it continued...for 'just a little more'. Until a year later it was done. And I had won.

~~~~~~~~~~~~~~~~~~~~

Diane Karchner

✽ ✽ ✽ ✽

Nausea

Nothing can prepare anyone for the nausea caused by the poison of chemotherapy agents coursing through your body. Nothing.

I had chemo twice a month, every month for two years. Forty-eight Wednesdays over two years I left work at noon, went to my doctor's office, got my injection (no pic or ports in 1973!), and made it home just in time. Never once did I get home too late. The anxiety of running into traffic gridlock or getting into an accident or some other weird holdup on the way home was overwhelming. I remember the turn onto that last street before ours — Blackman Street — only a mile more to go. The rumblings in my stomach always seemed to start with that turn. I hit the bathroom floor just in time. I always got to puke in private. That in itself has got to be some kind of miracle.

The first waves of nausea were accompanied by vomiting, just to make sure when the dry heaves started that there would be nothing but acid to burn my throat. Nausea like this was not just an uncomfortable, heartburn-y feeling. It rippled from my feet to the top of my head producing nothing but gagging and cold sweats and cramping. For hours. The dull headache that felt like a pressure bandage wrapped around my head lasted a couple of days longer.

Without effective prevention of this side effect, as many as 20% of patients postponed or even refused potentially curative treatment because of it.[64] With the introduction in the late 1970s of the extremely potent chemotherapy agent, cisplatin, nausea and vomiting soon became two of the most severe problems for patients treated with chemotherapy.[65]

The need was real.

Conducted in the 1960s, the first study in chemotherapy-induced nausea and vomiting (CINV) involved 300 patients with advanced gastric cancer hospitalized to receive their chemo treatment.[66] In the 1970s, more anti-nausea studies tested promising drugs.[67] Those studies, performed decades ago, led to the development of more than a half dozen effective treatments for CINV available today.

With their correct use, CINV can be prevented in up to 80% of all patients on chemotherapy.[68] To assist with proper administration of these drugs, the American Society of Clinical Oncology (OSCO) published the first CINV treatment guidelines in 1999, which has been updated in 2006.[69]

---

[64] http://theoncologist.alphamedpress.org/content/12/9/1143.full

[65] http://www.ncbi.nlm.nih.gov/pubmed/24157984

[66] https://www.moffitt.org/File%20Library/Main%20Nav/Research%20and%20Clinical%20Trials/Cancer%20Control%20Journal/v19s2/3.pdf

[67] https://www.moffitt.org/File%20Library/Main%20Nav/Research%20and%20Clinical%20Trials/Cancer%20Control%20Journal/v19s2/3.pdf

[68] http://www.ncbi.nlm.nih.gov/pubmed/24157984

[69] Kris MG, Hesketh PJ, Somerfield MR, et al: American Society of Clinical Oncology guideline for antiemetics in oncology: Update 2006. J Clin Oncol 24:2932-2947, 2006

If these drugs had been around in 1973, I would have had them in a candy dish on my coffee table.

Being a child of the wild and crazy '60's, I have kept my eye on the research surrounding the use of marijuana for CINV. Several controlled clinical trials have been performed supporting the beneficial effect of cannabinoids in the form of dronabinal (a manmade derivative of marijuana) which was approved by the FDA in 1985 for the treatment of CINV.[70] Even though approved, dronabinol (also known as Marinol)[71] has never proven to be as effective in clinical use as the newer CINV drugs, but it is still interesting to see non-pharmaceutical solutions investigated to solve medical challenges.

At present, there is insufficient evidence to recommend inhaling *cannabis* — that is, smoking a joint — as a treatment for cancer-related symptoms so there will be no toking on a doobie instead of sitting on the bathroom floor puking into a toilet. I have often joked about being a bald pothead with a smile on her face if this had proven true (and, *of course*, been made legally available!).

You never know what the future in research will hold. Science and curiosity-driven researchers continue to astound with their dedication to making things better, for pushing the boundaries of what is, to what can be — a cure for cancer.

~~~~~~~~~~~~~~~~~~~~~

---

[70] http://www.medicinenet.com/dronabinol-oral/article.htm

[71] http://www.medicinenet.com/dronabinol-oral/article.htm

Diane Karchner

❀ ❀ ❀ ❀

The Neck of the Hairless

Shining, gleaming, streaming, flaxen, waxen'. Flow it, show it, long as God can grow it, my hair. ~ Hair, The Cowsills, 1969

Today a bald head could mean a lot of things. For men, it could be a fashion statement or it could be a giving in to the receding hairline of aging. For women, it might be the same, but more likely it is not for attracting attention or dealing with life's aging eventualities. Today, as in 1973, baldness is usually a sign of illness. And of treatment. Today, it is a sign of hope that something is being done, something that just might work.

A question and answer page on OncoLink, the University of Pennsylvania's patient site, provides some level of understanding of why hair is lost in chemotherapy.

Chemotherapy kills both cancerous cells and other normal cells in your body. The normal cells in your body that are most at risk for being killed by chemotherapy are those that are growing at a fast rate. Because the cells responsible for hair growth are dividing at a rapid rate, they are sometimes destroyed by chemotherapy.[72]

Understanding it doesn't change the fact that it happens. And it happens regularly. More than the lack of hair, I notice the neck of a bald woman. There is something about the way a woman carries

---

[72] http://www.oncolink.org/experts/article.cfm?id=1057

herself when her head is cancer-bald. Proud. Courageous. Hopeful. Willing to put it out there for all to see. Maybe cover it a bit with a scarf or hat, maybe not. But out there for all to see.

I notice bald heads because I once had one. But I didn't feel courageous or proud or brave. It just wasn't how I felt in 1973. It wasn't how any of the baldies felt in 1973. My neck was more bowed, less proud, less courageous. I felt shame and embarrassment. Yup, I hear your screams. But it was the reality of the time. In 1973, baldness was no badass-giving-a-finger-to-cancer. No one shaved their own head in support of my fight for life. My baldness didn't pull people closer to me, it pushed them away. My baldness was not a badge of courage or hope; it was a mantle of sickness and disease and, mostly, death.

~~~~~~~~~~~~~~~~~~~~

I have lost some friends but many
relationships have become stronger.
I am a much better and more understanding
friend and parent. ~Laurie, Under Treatment

~~~~~~~~~~~~~~~~~~~~

Sounds so dramatic. It was. Every time I left the house I put myself on a darkened stage, yearning for notice and even some applause to encourage my fight. Instead, the audience walked out. The critics didn't even review the play. It was just never talked about. The cancer battle was like that — an off-off-off-Broadway show with a long run but no audience. This tragic drama played out in the lives of anyone who went through chemotherapy. Baldies. It told the world that we might die; there wasn't much need to pay attention since we would be gone soon.

A wig gave me a chance to pretend I was ok, and would be ok, and it didn't matter that the world might look at me funny with it perched precariously on my slippery head. The only wigs available in 1973 were 'fashion wigs.' There were no clinical or therapeutic reasons to buy a wig, and the quality and wig styles certainly reflected that notion — fluffy, curly, platinum, nets of glued on strands of synthetic 'hair,' with hard plastic combs to 'latch it' onto your own hair.

There was no 'fitting' of a wig. One size pretty much fit all, or was supposed to. I think the wig probably sat much stiller on heads with hair to 'latch' on to, but bald heads are slippery, so it slid around a bit. No, it slid around all the time, causing me to be in constant tug-and-pull acrobatics. Needless to say, it surely didn't look natural. But it served its purpose. People didn't have to look at my bald head. They were able to make eye contact without turning away. It was more for them than it was for me.

There were no organizations that helped with this.[73] No one donated hair in order to make the wigs more 'natural.'[74] No cool scarves or hats.[75] You and your bald head were on their own. Totally.

---

[73] http://www.cancerandcareers.org/en/at-work/where-to-start/Managing-Treatment-Side-Effects/Wigs-for-Cancer-Patients

[74] http://www.locksoflove.org/get-involved/

[75] https://www.tlcdirect.org/Cancer-Scarves-and-kerchiefs-for-Women-Cancer-and-Chemo-Patients-American-Cancer-Society-TLC-Direct

Sometimes, I think it was the baldness, not the cancer, that left me different, more guarded, less willing to put myself out there for anything or anyone. Still optimistic, still smiling, but inside I weighed every interaction, every eye contact. Even when my hair grew back, even when there were no outward signs of illness, I still didn't trust easily. I still assumed that no one cared enough to get through the uncomfortableness — the other bald places in my insides — to get to know me. Beyond what they saw. Even when my hair returned, trust never did.

In my blossoming pre-cancer faith, I had always really wanted God to come through with some thicker hair for me. But he didn't. Instead I got cancer and lost all of the little I had. I figured he was paying more attention to healing my body than whether or not I had hair on my head. Or maybe he was paying attention to all of it. Because a funny thing happened on the way back from baldness to hairy. My hair, although still not 's*hining, gleaming, streaming, flaxen, waxen'*, grew back thicker than it had ever been.

Ironic, right? God is funny that way.

~~~~~~~~~~~~~~~~~~~~~~

Remembering The Trembling

1973 was the beginning of the upsurge in breakthroughs for so many cancers, mine being right up front on that trek forward. But, even though my survival was still rare, I didn't talk about it. You would imagine I would want to, right? A victory of that magnitude. I beat the 'C' word when few others had! As cancers started to herald cures, curiosity and questioning started to be ok. Cancer stopped being so scary. It became less deadly. People would ask. Well-meaning people.

But for me, it was never a topic that I was willing to address. For me, it had happened and it was over. Done. I avoided everything about my cancer. I avoided talking about the triumph. I avoided discussing the medical breakthroughs. I avoided talking to doctors about it. I glossed over it when new doctors saw 'cancer' checked on my intake form. When asked by friends, I gave a quick answer then made a joke to deflect the conversation away from me. Or more specifically, away from my cancer.

~~~~~~~~~~~~~~~~~~~

It is something that happens but never goes away.
~ Kathy, In Treatment

~~~~~~~~~~~~~~~~~~~

Whether I talked about it or not, my insides reacted. Not violently, nothing that anyone could detect. But my insides, every inch of them, trembled. Imagine just narrowly missing being in a serious car accident. Your body is tingling with adrenaline rushing through the veins and arteries. You may be in a cold sweat, breathing fast, heart racing, stomach gurgling.

That's what I felt like every time I had to talk about cancer. Every time. Every single time. For years and years.

I have to admit, this was something I haven't thought much about since it stopped happening so much. So as I started research for this book, I thought it would be an area worth exploring, fully expecting that it would be a weird Diane-thing and not a shared experience by other survivors. I was wrong.

Post-traumatic stress disorder (PTSD) is an anxiety disorder, developing after experiencing an extremely frightening or life-threatening situation. Most often associated with traumatic events such as war, sexual and physical attacks, natural disasters, and serious accidents, it can also affect people with a history of cancer.[76]

In 1994, the American Psychiatric Association redefined its trauma criteria for the diagnosis of PTSD to include life-threatening illness, like cancer.[77] NCI studies confirm that 3%-4% of patients with early stage cancer, and as many as 35% of patients evaluated after treatment, meet full or partial PTSD criteria. Not surprising, the research also indicates as many as 80% of patients diagnosed with recurrence may

---

[76] http://www.cancer.net/survivorship/life-after-cancer/post-traumatic-stress-disorder-and-cancer

[77] http://www.medscape.com/viewarticle/708048

have some level of PTSD symptoms.[78] Additionally, a recent study found that nearly 1 in 4 women who were newly diagnosed with breast cancer experienced PTSD.[79]

This isn't just a Diane-thing. This is a cancer-thing.

PTSD symptoms are different for each person. They can come and go with the symptoms. Usually developing within three months of the cancer diagnosis, they can also occur several months or even years later.[80]

~~~~~~~~~~~~~~~~~~~~

I had a lot of support during cancer and
I was so grateful for that but I really struggled more
in the years following cancer. Friends and family
moved on and I suppose I didn't. I felt very alone.
I battled severe depression for a few years. I think t
he most difficult days of cancer were the years
following treatment. ~Jennifer, Cancer Survivor

~~~~~~~~~~~~~~~~~~~~

The symptoms I experienced were explained well in this 1999 study: 'Defining symptoms include trauma-associated dreams and nightmares, efforts to avoid reminders of the stressful experience, and

---

[78] Knobf, 2007; NCI; Shelby, Golden-Kreutz, & Andersen, 2008).[http://www.medscape.com/viewarticle/708048_3

[79] http://www.cancer.net/survivorship/life-after-cancer/post-traumatic-stress-disorder-and-cancer

[80] http://www.cancer.net/survivorship/life-after-cancer/post-traumatic-stress-disorder-and-cancer

heightened physiologic arousal.'[81] Fortunately, I never had bad dreams or nightmares related to the cancer. But I did avoid any reminder of it, and I've certainly had a physiologic response when reminded of it (like when writing about it!).

I was never diagnosed with PTSD. In 1973 doctors were not looking for it and patients didn't mention it — including me. Although not everyone experiences this as a result of a cancer diagnosis or treatment, today there is a high level of awareness by all in the oncology field of the high risk for psychological and social consequences with the diagnosis and treatment of cancer. Cancer-induced PTSD is not a singular event. Its effect is not always short-lived. It could extend from diagnosis into survivorship, possibly lasting a whole lifetime.[82]

Today an entire field of study, called psycho-oncology, is dedicated to the psychological impact of cancer on a patient. This specialty field in cancer care is 'concerned with understanding and treating the social, psychological, emotional, spiritual, quality-of-life and functional aspects of cancer, from prevention through bereavement. It is a whole-person approach to cancer care that addresses a range of very human needs that can improve quality of life for people affected by cancer.'[83]

---

[81] Smith M., et.al. Validation of PTSD Checklist. J Trauma Stress. July 1999, v12.3. pp485-499

[82] http://www.medscape.com/viewarticle/708048_3

[83] http://www.capo.ca/patient-family-resources/what-is-psychosocial-oncology/

~~~~~~~~~~~~~~~~~~~~

I don't actually believe that anyone can ever
know that they are "cured" of cancer. I think most
people are just in remission or NED - often for
years or even a life-time. ~Laurie, Under Treatment

~~~~~~~~~~~~~~~~~~~~

Today's cancer patients may have a much lower risk of PTSD than I did, particularly if they have good social support, clear information about the stage of their cancer, and an open relationship with their oncology team.[84] I had no social support except my immediate family. I had little or no information about the stage of my cancer since there was so little available. But I did have a relationship with my team — that is, the one member, my doctor, and he had the few answers available at the time.

~~~~~~~~~~~~~~~~~~~~

---

[84] http://www.cancer.gov/about-cancer/coping/survivorship/new-normal/ptsd-pdq

Diane Karchner

❀ ❀ ❀ ❀

Lone Survivor

Once I got through chemo, I realized there was a lot of work to be done to support others with this diagnosis. I wanted to help. The only organization in our area, or almost anywhere, that seemed to be doing anything was the American Cancer Society. So I called the local chapter and was put in touch with a woman who was leading the local fundraiser. Big ticket dinner event. It sounded exciting. So I attended the planning meeting.

It was in, shall we say, a better area of town than I was used to. Not to say I was intimidated by the wealthy, but I can say that I was way, way out of my comfort zone. The women (and it was only women) held their teacups in a way I had never thought to (I only owned mugs). They drank martinis out of glasses with long, elegant stems (I only drank beer out of a can or wine with a twist-off cap). They dressed really nice for an evening meeting (I had on frayed bell-bottom jeans and a gauzy peasant shirt).

Nope, none of that made me uncomfortable. Nope, I was fine. Not. To be perfectly honest, the only thing about them that did not intimidate me was that they were all twenty-five years older than me. At least, on that score, I thought I was the winner.

No matter what level of intimidation I struggled with, the women were gracious and nice and since they all knew each other well, I was the only one asked to introduce myself. So I did. Which I did well. I did.

I said 'I came to find out how I could help raise money for cancer, because I had it, and now I don't.' Eloquent, confident and coherent.

Ah, not.

What I actually mumbled was *'I had cancer.'* Period.

My post-traumatic tremors started almost immediately. My stomach began its usual rollover. But I took a deep breath and smiled through it, uncomfortable with my own words as much as with the sudden stillness in the room. It was like everything had been suspended in a slow motion time warp. The caterer (yes, they had one!) stopped refreshing the beverage cart. The fire in the hearth seemed relieved of all oxygen. No one seemed to move.

I thought for years that their reaction was because they didn't like me. They never asked any more questions, never engaged me in a personal conversation again. It was like I hadn't said anything of importance, that I said I came to the meeting because the sky was blue.

It was years later that I finally figured it out. These gracious women weren't involved in the American Cancer Society because they were just being altruistic. They were doing it because they had each lost a loved one to cancer. And there in front of them sat someone who had made it, who had survived. A stranger. A hippie girl with stringy, thin blond hair and a see-through blouse. She had made it and my <insert

loved one's name> had not. They had never met a survivor. It caught them by surprise.

If I had been a more intuitive twenty-something I would have felt survivor remorse coming on strong, but I hadn't even fully accepted my own survival yet, so it was hard to get my head around those who hadn't. I wasn't in a place where I was sorry that I did, sorry that others did not. I was just there, trembling inside. It was a confusing state of suspended animation.

Cancer was in so many ways a solo disease. A singular sport. Just as there was no team surrounding you as you as you fought the good fight, there was no one to help you process through your survival. Today it is different in so many ways. The American Cancer Society has the Cancer Survivor Network (CSN) created solely for survivors to talk to each other, a safe place to share concerns and fears. Its site description clearly highlights what had been so lacking: "Create your own personal space to tell us about yourself and your cancer experience, share photos, audio, etc., start an online journal, contribute resources, and more. Expressing feelings and experiences and supporting one another is what CSN is all about."[85]

Recently, a public awareness campaign began in the media, sponsored by the Entertainment Industry Foundation. The campaign is called StandUP2Cancer,[86] with a tagline of 'It's impossible to beat

---

[85] http://csn.cancer.org

[86] http://www.standup2cancer.org/mission_statement

cancer. Alone.' The first time I saw the ad I was only in outline form of this book, so I gave it little attention.

But halfway through this chapter I opened a newspaper to a full-page ad with that tagline staring me in the face. It took my breath away. The rest of the ad expanded on the thought of not battling this alone: 'It takes all of us to beat cancer. Doctors, researchers, volunteers and most importantly, people like you. Join the movement to beat cancer.' This kind of media hype and awareness-generation encourages those with cancer. It has to.

~~~~~~~~~~~~~~~~~~~~

While I was fighting cancer, my family and friends
were amazing. They all rallied around me and
were incredibly loving and supportive. I tell people
that it was one of the blessings of cancer. It was like
getting to be at my own funeral because
I got to hear all the good things that people think
about me. My relationships with my friends and
family were strengthened by my experience.
~Kim, Cancer Survivor

~~~~~~~~~~~~~~~~~~~~

Others are pouring dollars and time and influence into beating cancer, for good. The pink ribbon campaign, specifically the Susan B. Komen[87] walk/run for breast cancer, is perhaps the best known of all.

---

[87] http://ww5.komen.org/AboutUs/OurWork.html

In 1982, the pink ribbon was used solely for breast cancer awareness, worn by runners in a race in New York City. By 1990, the pink ribbon expanded from just awareness to include survivorship, with women who had survived breast cancer — and there weren't many of them then — honored with special ribbons and visors to wear during the race/walk, now expanded to major cities across the country. Originally started to raise awareness of the number of women dying from this cancer, millions of dollars are now poured into research to get to the cure. Think of how far the research and treatment regimens for breast cancer have come in those years.

For those of us who remember years like 1973, all of this could leave a sour taste of neglect in our mouths, until we remember what it was really like to feel that abandoned. For me, I am overwhelmed with thankfulness that my younger friends who have faced the aloneness of the cancer diagnosis, are well-supported and noticed as they move to survivor mode.

But I will go back to a comment from the blog I mentioned earlier. "Cancer has caused us all pain and its only remedy is banding together to support our mutual healing."[88]

We can't feel too harshly of the medical community of decades ago, or that others hadn't thought to develop support groups or initiatives like StandUp2Cancer or Pink ribbon'd events.

---

[88] http://www.wherewegonow.com/debbies_blog/cancer-survivors-guilt-its-ugly-cousin

In 1973, cancer was burying more than were surviving. Many more. They were barely keeping people alive, let alone dealing with or even noticing what the survivors were going through.

Those many years ago, I was just a young woman, sitting in a living room, trying to come to grips with survival, to help. And those ladies were just trying to cope with their loss.

No one knew what to do with those who made it through.

Not yet.

~~~~~~~~~~~~~~~~~~~~

Not A Hero For Life

I end up where I began. I survived.

My sister did not. And the hope that will no longer be.

Hope.

Hope is a funny thing. Defined as 'a feeling of expectation and desire for a certain thing to happen.' It can exist in a vacuum or in a whirlwind of chaos. It can get you through exciting, positive times. It can give you a positive outlook when things are going bad.

~~~~~~~~~~~~~~~~~~

Cling to hope. I had no idea chaplains
could be so helpful,
ask for one if you need to talk!
~ Jennifer, Cancer Survivor

~~~~~~~~~~~~~~~~~~

I hoped that my cancer would go away. I hoped that the chemo would work. I hoped that I would get home after the injection before I started vomiting. Hope gave me something to be positive about, to look forward to.

But hope was more than just wishing things would happen, and happen well. It was an underlying belief that eventually life would return to normal, that I would bounce back better than ever. It was a deep desire for normal to prevail.

~~~~~~~~~~~~~~~~~~~~~

Be focused, be joyful. You never know when
your last day on earth is. It could be you walk
outside and get struck by lightening,
a flying object out of nowhere or a car, and that
could be it. It may not be the cancer at all.
So, live each day fully — say I'm sorry,
I love you and I forgive you.
~Nancy, Cancer Survivor

~~~~~~~~~~~~~~~~~~~~~

University of Connecticut psychologist Keith Bellizzi wrote that some life events are so intense that many people use them to reconstruct their lives; they don't return to the same level of functioning but to a greater level. "Post-traumatic growth is above and beyond resilience. Life after cancer means finding a new normal, but for many the new normal is better than the old normal."[89]

For me, the change wasn't dramatic, it couldn't really be seen by different career or life choices, by taking up a new hobby, or taking on more sky-diving-type risks. Even though I was no longer belly-baring, I basically looked the same to most people. Yet something had changed. Inside. My perspective on my old normal changed. It was

---

[89] https://www.psychologytoday.com/articles/200907/the-new-survivors

more thankful, more appreciative of the little things, of the people. I was still feisty and opinionated (my family may see that as an understatement), yet calmer in some way.

~~~~~~~~~~~~~~~~~~~~~~

I was the beneficiary of many kind acts
by friends and acquaintances
when going through treatment.
That has made me become more aware of
how even little acts can truly impact someone's
life. So I no longer question if
I should help (fearing what I do may be
insignificant or might hinder) when I
see a friend in need, I just do it.
~Kendra, cancer in remission

~~~~~~~~~~~~~~~~~~~~~~

Citing two decades of research, a 2014 article in Psychology Today referred to this state of uncommon calm when people who have been through a traumatic event, like cancer, change their perspective as they move forward. This involves the building of life's choices on a firm understanding of reality, rather than on the past trauma. "This is more realistic than simple positivity yet more positive than pessimism. We like to call this grounded hope, an approach involving building one's choices on a firm understanding of reality."[90]

---

[90] https://www.psychologytoday.com/articles/201406/super-survival-the-fittest

Maybe that word sums it up: reality. I have a more realistic view of the problems and trauma of normal life. After all, I might have lost the battle with cancer. But I didn't. So what could life throw at me that was bigger and stronger and more terrifying than dying from cancer? This new normal was hard fought.

~~~~~~~~~~~~~~~~~~~~~~~

Find something to laugh hearty about every day.

Believe in tomorrow.

~Grace, 'currently cancer-free'

~~~~~~~~~~~~~~~~~~~~~~~

Which brings me to a hard topic. Heroism.

I believe that everyone who has been through cancer — and those still fighting on — are heroes in their fight. I do, with all my heart. I can truthfully say I would have considered myself a kind of hero while I was in the throes of treatment. But I have read and heard and watched cancer survivors raised to a lifetime hero status. And, as a survivor, I do not agree.

Now before you scream at me, hold on.

A hero is defined as someone who is admired for her courage. Heroes don't think they have a different choice other than the seemingly heroic one they made. A hero, whether running into battle or sitting in an infusion chair for an hour every week, sees no other way than the way forward, into the mayhem and danger and pain for a cause greater and grander than doing nothing.

The problem is when hero status becomes a life-long claim, a life-long descriptor. I am not a hero today, in my normal, daily life. I do not run into a firestorm every day to slay the dragon, in fact, I avoid some if I can help it. I am not fighting impossible odds every morning that I awake. I am a normal person, living life a day at a time. Perhaps changed by my battle, by my heroic choices borne out by pain-induced battle scars. But I am no hero. I believe that most survivors would agree.

My nephew served in the Army, doing three tours in battle zones across the Middle East. I believe, although he talks rarely in details, he was a hero during those months in the war zones. I would wager that he walked into danger, went beyond the normal to serve and defend. He, and his fellow soldiers, are honored when they return, saluted in airports, treated to meals in restaurants. I think they should be. Until they are not. Today, out of uniform, he would not consider himself a hero by any means.

Hero is a state of mind. If faced with the same kind of difficulty, same kind of battle, a hero would rise up again and slay that dragon. Heroism is a state of mind that a hero does not appreciate or own when he is trudging through the hero-inducing battle. A hero does what has to be done, then moves on.

The problem arises when the hero state of mind is accepted as the normal. When someone accepts the title of hero, absorbs it into his self-image, creating a false sense of power and misplaced self-grandeur They place a halo on their head as a normal part of their daily dress. With this halo acceptance, that hero status is who you are rather than what you did. If it persists, it can destroy, like it did with Lance Armstrong. We saw him as a hero who physically, bravely, almost super-humanly fought through cancer. It was a rare and public display of heroism, worthy of celebration and applause. Inspirational. It was. But much of his troubles later in life may have come from that halo getting too tight, feeling it needed to be earned over and over, no matter what it took.[91]

Yet a man like John McCain, although applauded for his endurance and his heroism as a prisoner of war, leans on who he is today, not what he had done in the past. Yes, we know of his heroic acts. Yet we can see him as a political figure who did heroic acts years ago, not as a hero who is a politician. He does not need to prove his heroism over and over again. He is not running into burning buildings so we will choose him at the voting polls.

~~~~~~~~~~~~~~~~~~~~~

I just wanted to get things moving, do what
I needed to do, surgery, chemo and move on.
~ Stacey, Breast Cancer Survivor

~~~~~~~~~~~~~~~~~~~~~

We were not created, as humans, to exist with the mantle of hero. We were not created to be put on a pedestal, to be admired forever for

---

[91] https://www.psychologytoday.com/blog/supersurvivors/201301/zero-worship-did-surviving-cancer-make-armstrong-hero

one hard-won battle. It's too hard to balance up there and live a normal life.

Cancer survivors do not want to be called heroes. They appreciate being encouraged, supported, admired for the bravery it took to move another step into the pain that could lead to health. Survivors want to get back to life, rather than slog through the recalls and memories of past battles, of past heroics, of the trembling of remembering. Survivors, for the most part, don't want the halo of hero. They would rather move on and be applauded for being alive, for getting back to life, escaping the limbo world of cancer wars.

Hope is not in the hero halo.

Hope is in life.

That someday there will be a normal life.

Again.

~~~~~~~~~~~~~~~~~~~~~~

Diane Karchner

❀ ❀ ❀ ❀

What's Love Got to Do With It?

I lived on hope those seven years. I trusted that hope would not fail me, that what I hoped for would come to pass. Hope is different from faith, yet there can be no faith until you have hope that something, someone, will come through.

Hope wishes for it. Faith is knowing it will.

I wasn't a faith-filled, spiritual person when I was diagnosed with cancer in 1973. My life with God had been peppered with a shallow faith that he existed, that he had something in mind for me, someday. I believed that he loved me. But I believed that when it came to my daily life, for my daily struggles, that I was alone.

A couple of years later, I found Jesus - or rather he found me.

I say it that way because I believe that God pursues us. Steadily, smoothly, constantly. He never gives up on any of us, not one. Because he loves us that much.

Anne Lamott, in her memoir of faith, *Traveling Mercies*,[92] told this story of God's pursuit that has remained with me for years.

> *After a while, as I lay there, I became aware of someone with me, hunkered down in the corner. The feeling was so strong that I actually turned on the light for a moment to make sure no one was*

---

[92] http://www.amazon.com/Traveling-Mercies-Some-Thoughts-Faith/dp/0385496095?ie=UTF8&keywords=anne%20lamott&qid=1461809431&ref_=sr_1_5&sr=8-5

there – of course, there wasn't. But after a while, in the dark again, I knew beyond any doubt that it was Jesus. I felt him as surely as I feel my dog lying nearby as I write this. I felt him just sitting there on his haunches in the corner of my sleeping loft, watching me with patience and love, and I squinched my eyes shut, but that didn't help because that's not what I was seeing him with.

Faith in God wasn't my problem when I went through cancer treatment. Faith in Jesus was what I had been missing. God is God. He's dang big, hard to grasp, and harder still to think he might care enough about little old me. But then he came to earth, walked and talked and healed and prayed. He was a human, in the flesh. And that made God, for us weak and flawed humans, easier to grab hold of.

And I did. Once I believed that Jesus is God, it became easier to grasp a real faith. He died, rose again, and is alive and well and listening to my every whine, watching my every move, and flooding me with love and forgiveness. It is a hard thing to run away from, a hard thing to dispute. It's a balm to the soul.

~~~~~~~~~~~~~~~~~~~~

I have had to rely very heavily in my faith that
God is in control in what most days feels like a
very out of control situation. ~Debbie, In Treatment

~~~~~~~~~~~~~~~~~~~~

I often think what those few years with the cancer fight might have been like if I had the faith I have today. More than grounded hope.

More than just a desire to get through it. With faith, I would have really known that all was going to be OK.

Faith like that doesn't mean that I was guaranteed a cure. Faith like that doesn't mean that treatment was going to be easy, that the nausea was never going to happen. Faith like that meant that I was never alone and that everything was going to work out. Some how. Faith like that is a trust issue. And I have learned to trust that God will work everything out for good, for real good. Eventually.

Because he loves us. Each of us.

~~~~~~~~~~~~~~~~~~~

For the first few years God and I didn't speak.

I still have issues but I am better now then before.

~Shana, Cancer Survivor

~~~~~~~~~~~~~~~~~~~

1st Corinthians chapter 13, the chapter of the Bible so often read at weddings, is thirteen verses of the love that God has for us, the kind of love we are to have for each other. I love all the words in this passage, its description of a love that transcends everything. Kind, gentle.

But there in one verse in that passage that has always stuck with me, giving me an often uncomfortable standard to live with.

If I have a faith that moves mountains, but have not love, I gain nothing. ~1 Corinthians 13.3

Without love, I gain absolutely nothing of any importance, of any worth. Love is a powerful elixir to our hurts and our wounds, but it's also a powerful way to live. With love, nothing, absolutely nothing, goes to waste. Everything we do for each other in love, has some value. To you, to the one you are loving on, to God. He wants us to live this vast, borderless way of love.

If I had to do things differently, if I had something to change (other than not getting cancer), I always thought I would want to have gone through the cancer knowing Jesus, having him by my side. That's what I have wished for, but perhaps that is exactly where he wanted me to be, learning the difference between having him or not. Being alone, or not. Relying too much on me, rather than him.

~~~~~~~~~~~~~~~~~~~~

I was raised in the church, however a 20-year career
in Fire/EMS had changed my views on God,
and I had fallen out of faith. However, when they
rolled me onto the BMT unit, the world
came crashing in. I cried to my mom, and said,
"I can't do this mom, I'm not strong enough."
(Which even typing this makes me tear up.)
So we prayed on it, and I instantly felt better. Even throughout
almost a year of treatment, I've always felt calm.
~Benjamin, Cancer Survivor

~~~~~~~~~~~~~~~~~~~~

Funny thing is I was wanting something that was already there. He was there. He was always there. Every second. When I got the diagnosis. When I struggled after surgery. When I laid on the bathroom floor with nausea that rocked my body. Every day of that two years of treatment. He was there, as Anne Lamott so beautifully described, 'hunkered down in the corner.'

Even when I didn't talk to him, didn't believe in him, didn't want to have anything to do with him, he was there. We can't get rid of the guy no matter what. He will not leave us, ever. That means never. From birth to beyond death (for believers), he is by our side. Waiting for us to choose him. Waiting for us to choose love.

~~~~~~~~~~~~~~~~~~~~

Jesus never left my side! Through my cancer experience
I had the opportunity to mature in my faith.
~Cathy, Cancer Survivor

~~~~~~~~~~~~~~~~~~~~

If I don't have love, I have nothing. But if I have it, I have everything.

I have talked to survivors who have had Jesus in their lives as they moved through all that is cancer. It didn't change anything in their treatment. Their fears were still there. Their anguish and pain still raw and just below the surface. But they never felt alone. They always felt that they had someone in their corner to walk them through all of it.

Jesus isn't a magic elixir to take all of the hurts and hardships of our lives away, to make every aspect perfect and painless. He is there, in our lives, because he created us to love him, to bring him glory and praise because getting through this life — cancer or not — is dang hard on our own. He walked on the dirt of the earth. He knows how hard all this is.

I am so glad I know Jesus.

I am so glad he loves me so much that he never left me alone then, never leaves me alone now.

~~~~~~~~~~~~~~~~~~~~

My faith became stronger because that's how I got through the whole ordeal. ~Gina, Cancer Survivor

~~~~~~~~~~~~~~~~~~~~

And now these three remain: faith, hope and love. The greatest of these is love. ~1 Corinthians 13.13

~~~~~~~~~~~~~~~~~~~~

If There Was Ever a Time...

I wrote earlier that 1973 was the right-est time there could have been to have cancer. Before then, cure rates were horrid, and getting worse. Attention to research was on the back burner, if it was on the stove cooking at all.

1973 seemed to be that turning point, that moment in time when the momentum was reversed, when research and treatment breakthroughs accelerated, when the number of sure-deaths began to decline.

In 1973 there was less than a 50% 5-year survival rate, meaning that half of those who had cancer died within 5 years of diagnosis. For those who lived those 5 years, many of them died soon after. It looked bleak when I received my diagnosis.

Yet there was so much happening that I could not see, that I did not appreciate for its value to life and cures.

In 1971 the National Cancer Act accelerated everything, by pouring funding into cancer research and medical solutions.

In 1972 the subspecialty of oncology was approved for the first time. The medical community was noticing. Not that they hadn't noticed the killer disease before but they now were noticing that not all cancer diagnoses were death sentences. They knew there was hope on the horizon.

The CT Scanner was discovered in 1972. Not yet widely used until a few years later, it has become one of the diagnostic tools of choice for most oncologists today.

In 1973 Johns Hopkins Cancer Center opened its doors, one of the few in the country at the time, soon joined by dozens more within a few years.

Staging Hodgkins lymphoma by laparotomy was only demonstrated as successful in early 1973 — just months before my diagnosis.

In 1977, the medical community standardized the language to stage cancer tumors, enabling data, treatment and outcome sharing that had never been available before.

If there was ever a time for me to be diagnosed with cancer, that was the decade to do it. So much happening in the field of oncology. My treatment, as painful as they were, played a part in validating what would work, and what might not.

Today, a cancer diagnosis is not as automatic a death sentence as it used to be. 14.5 million people diagnosed with cancer are alive in 2016. More than half of those would probably have not survived in 1973. Maybe more.

Nausea is no longer a side effect that keeps people away from needed treatment.

Those who are susceptible to breast cancer can find out for sure, instead of living a life in fear of the unknown.

Remission, even if short-lived, is more common than ever. Longer survival means that time works in their favor. Research is so close to taking remission to cure.

The Human Genome Project, completed in 2003, opened the door for the development of immunotherapies that are using a patient's own cells to fight the cancer that is attacking.

In 2016, VP Biden's 'Moonshot to the Cure' project will infuse cancer research with needed funds to tip the scales.

As I was editing the last chapters of this book I got an email from a friend that a work colleague of ours had died of pancreatic cancer. Less than a year after diagnosis. It left me breathless and sad. Another loss.

Yet, this loss, this sadness used to be the norm, not the exception.

If there is ever a time for the hope of a cure for all cancers, it is now.

And what a celebration that will be.

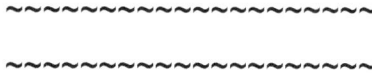

~~~~~~~~~~~~~~~~~~~~
~~~~~~~~~~~~~~~~~~~~

Diane Karchner

Diane Karchner

www.ingramcontent.com/pod-product-compliance
Lightning Source LLC
Chambersburg PA
CBHW060617210326
41520CB00010B/1373